Dr. Miriam Stoppard's
Pregnancy
and Birth Book

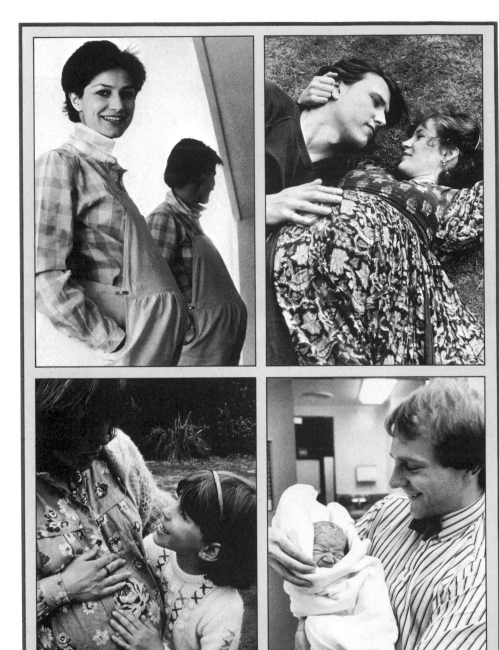

Dr. Miriam Stoppard's
Pregnancy
and Birth Book
Dr. Miriam Stoppard

PHOTOGRAPHY BY
Nancy Durrell McKenna

BALLANTINE BOOKS • NEW YORK

For my sister, Hazel

Originally published in the United Kingdom under the
title *The Pregnancy and Birth Book*.

Library of Congress Catalog Card Number: 86-91577

ISBN: 0-345-31908-7

This edition published by arrangement with
Villard Books.

Cover design by Wendy Bass and Richard Aquan,
photo by Tana Hoban.

Manufactured in the United States of America

First Ballantine Books Edition: July 1987

10 9 8 7 6

Contents

Introduction   6–11

Pregnancy calendar   12–21

1 Deciding to have a baby   22–33

2 Finding out you are pregnant   34–41

3 Choices in childbirth   42–57

4 Prenatal care   58–69

5 The growing baby   70–79

6 Physical changes   80–89

7 Emotional changes   90–95

8 Health and nutrition   96–107

9 Exercise   108–121

10 Looking good   122–127

11 Rest and relaxation   128–135

12 Common complaints   136–143

13 Special-care pregnancies   144–151

14 Preparing for the birth   152–159

15 Labor and birth   160–191

16 Complications of the birth   192–201

17 The first days   202–217

18 Getting back to normal   218–227

Appendix   228

Rights and benefits   228

Useful addresses   229–230

Further reading   231

Glossary   232–233

Index   234–239

Acknowledgements   240

Introduction

The subject of pregnancy is one I've written about for almost ten years and I was quite surprised when I came to write this book at how my own attitudes have changed since I first put pen to paper on the subject. I wrote then as though pregnancy was controlled by "givens." Furthermore, these "givens" were dictated by the medical profession. The fact that a woman might not want to have her baby in a hospital, might not want to have her perineum shaved, might want to have her partner or a friend with her during labor, was something that was outside the "givens" and therefore difficult to accommodate.

As I began to write this book I realized that all these preconceptions were gone. During the last ten years quite a revolution has taken place in the way we view pregnancy. Women have different attitudes towards childbirth, and doctors have a different approach to it. Pregnant women no longer see themselves as patients nor want to be treated as infirm. Doctors increasingly see pregnant women as healthy women who need medical care and support, which whenever possible should be tailor-made to suit the individual. Our attitudes to pregnancy are no longer prescriptive, they're to do with options and choices. What I have set out to do here is to give you information about the whys and wherefores of pregnancy, about what is absolutely necessary and what is not, about what is a matter of dogma and what is not, about techniques that are customary rather than essential and to show you where your areas of choice lie.

Pregnancy, labor and birth ought to be joyful experiences for a woman and her partner. Above all else I hope this book will help you both to feel really positive about pregnancy and birth. For this to happen, it is important to know that options do exist. Armed with this knowledge you will find the courage and enthusiasm to ask questions and get the information you need in order to exercise your options and make choices that suit you. It's not possible for you as a lay person to discuss the pros and cons of having to lie flat in the delivery room with a physician or midwife if you're not familiar with the mechanics of labor. Without some basic facts you cannot argue that it's much better for you to move around freely and stand up as long as you can during the first stage of labor. You cannot opt for an upright position in which to deliver the baby if you are unversed in the merits of this position.

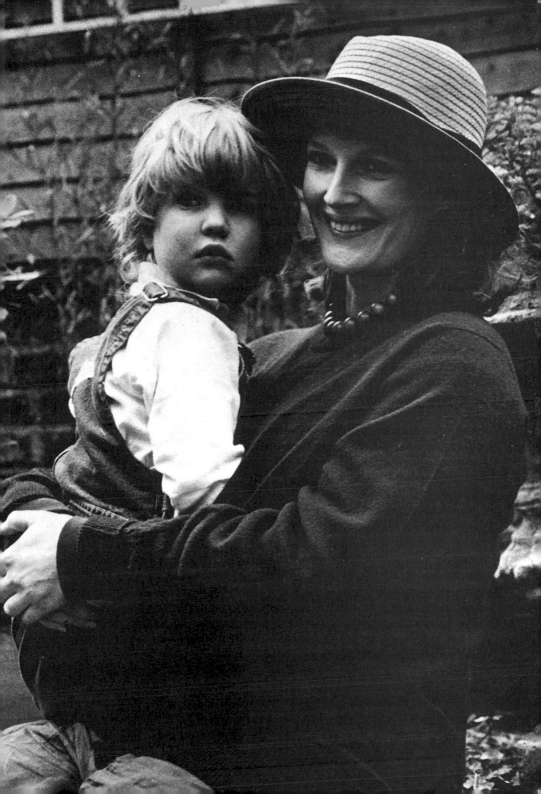

So this book aims to give you an outline of the options that lie before you, and then, having decided on the options that suit you, the courage to try to get the kind of delivery and birth you want. I have included not only useful information to help a couple to have a reasoned discussion with a doctor or nurse, but I have also given lists of possible questions to ask when choosing a hospital, and a suggested letter to write in order to get the birth of your choice.

My other aim is to remove fear and mystery by presenting information openly and objectively. It's been known for decades that fear of the unknown in pregnancy causes pain, discomfort and slow, difficult labors. If, on the other hand, a woman has been trained during her pregnancy to listen to and observe her body, to read its messages, to act with them and help them, particularly with breathing techniques, relaxation exercises and exercises for the pelvic muscles, she can greatly assist herself in shortening the birth, making it less painful, a great deal more comfortable and a truly joyful event.

Fathers

There is much research to show that if men are involved from the moment pregnancy is confirmed they become active and enthusiastic fathers. This means being involved in all the preparations, attendance at prenatal classes and visits, in decisions as to where and how to have the baby, and with the care of the baby from day one. If men are shut out at any stage, the role of father is more difficult to assimilate. There is no greater help to a pregnant woman than an interested and sympathetic partner. There is no better medical attendant in the delivery room than an understanding, supportive father. There is certainly no better help with a newborn baby than an active, passionate dad. The labor itself can be just as remarkable an experience for the father, as this letter testifies.

66 Regardless of where the baby is being born, at home or in the hospital, be prepared to leave your sense of embarrassment somewhere else – you will soon realize that what is happening to your wife is the most real thing she's ever experienced. She may groan and moan softly or loudly, become totally uninterested in

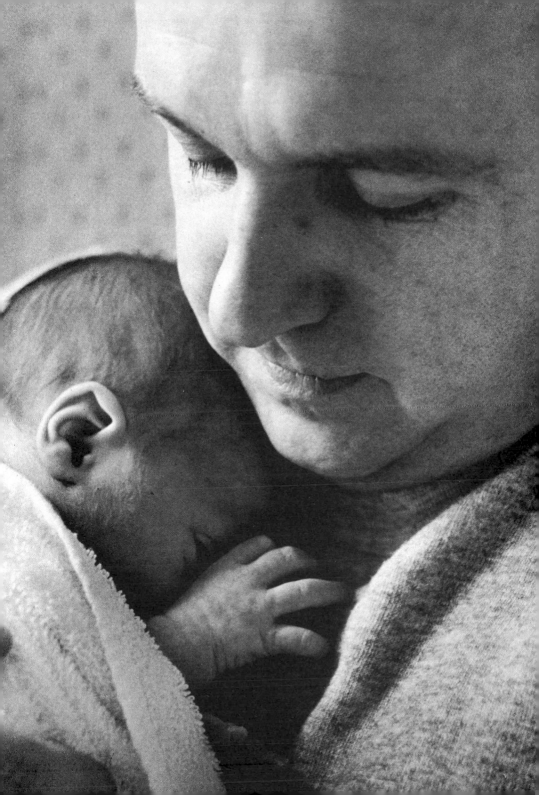

you, ask you questions you have no answers for ("How much longer?"). So since she's putting her whole self into the labor, it will help her and you if you become as totally involved as possible. You can help her greatly by answering the questions the nurses ask and by making the decisions – she's in no state to think about anything but what is happening to her body – and above all by being positive. Never cast even a shadow of doubt into her mind. Always tell her that she's doing well, because no matter what she is doing, she's doing the best she can. Do not judge her – help her, give her some of your energy. The amount of togetherness you discover during the birth of your child will remain with you and grow for the rest of your lives. **99**

A major priority for a pregnant woman is to have adequate help. While the best help may be a partner, it doesn't have to be. It may be more practical and even more emotionally supportive to have a close friend, of either sex, to be your birth assistant. An option you might like to exercise is having both your partner and a friend with you during labor. To clear this path necessitates long-term planning and involvement from the beginning for all concerned with your prenatal classes, and discussions with your doctor or midwife about how your labor will be conducted. As you can imagine this isn't always straightforward, but the book will help you to pick your way through various possibilities.

Approaching motherhood
In writing this book, I have also taken into account the fact that for many women today motherhood comes rather later in life than it used to. It's now commonplace for a woman to pursue her career into her thirties and decide to have her first child somewhere around 35. The old obstetric concept of being an "elderly" primipara after the age of 30 (or even after the age of 25) may have to be renamed simply because it is becoming so common. Doctors are now used to dealing with first-time mothers in the older age groups and see it as a normal event rather than a cause for alarm. At one time the medical profession suspected that every mother over 30 would have problems. We now know that these problems are hardly more common than in younger women.

Most women opt to work for at least part of their pregnancy. This means that the planning for a modern pregnancy and the birth is quite different from that in the past when many women left work and stayed at home until they became pregnant. Now most women feel they have to give careful consideration to their future job security. With this in mind, I have outlined the advantages and disadvantages of combining work, pregnancy and motherhood. Even if you have decided to resume your job after, say, six months, you may find it impossible to leave your baby and decide to wait for a few months longer. No one knows before the birth of their own child just how they will feel in the event. As more and more women are opting to work it is important to think about how this situation can be eased.

Every woman is beset by doubts, fears and anxieties – you would not be normal if you did not have them. Yet it will all seem easy and straightforward in retrospect. In the meantime, it's reassuring to think about the women all around you, hardly different from yourself, who are enjoying pregnancies, having memorable labors and births and, despite some sleepless nights, worries about feedings and weight gain, are thrilled with their babies. They find that pregnancy and birth introduce them to a fulfilling phase of their lives.

Miriam Stoppard

Pregnancy calendar

Knowing about the changes inside you during pregnancy helps you to become more aware of your body and its needs. This week-by-week calendar of the development of the baby and the changes in your body summarizes the information so that you'll be better equipped to understand what is happening to you in your pregnancy and to enjoy it. As no two pregnancies develop at the same rate, don't be alarmed if you haven't experienced or noticed certain changes; they will come in time.

Signs of pregnancy

You may know or suspect that you are pregnant from one or more of the following signs:
- missed period
- feeling nauseous
- change in taste and preference for certain foods
- metallic taste in your mouth
- changes in your breasts
- frequency of urination
- tiredness
- increase in vaginal discharge

Pregnancy tests

- The most common means of pregnancy testing is the detection of a certain hormone in your urine (see p. 36). You can either go to your doctor, or buy a home kit and test the urine yourself. This test is not 100 per cent reliable until at least two weeks after the first day of your missed period.
- A blood test will reveal pregnancy hormones even before your first missed period.
- An internal examination by your doctor will confirm pregnancy by the eighth week after the first day of your last period.

Duration of pregnancy

In this book, pregnancy is dated from day 1 of your last menstrual period (see p. 37). If you have an average 28-day cycle, fertilization is counted as taking place around day 14 and not day 1 of your pregnancy. This timescale allows that pregnancy, which actually lasts some 266 days from fertilization, continues for 40 weeks.

WEEKS 3–4

Estrogen and progesterone levels increase steadily following fertilization of the ovum, producing changes in your body's structure and metabolism so that you can support and nourish your developing baby.

The blastocyst produces enough hormone (HCG) to maintain pregnancy. Implants itself in the lining of the womb.

WEEKS 4–5

Menstruation is suppressed, though some women do experience breakthrough bleeding.

- If you suspect you are pregnant, stop taking any medication and check with your doctor.
- Stop smoking and drinking alcohol. If you can't completely, cut back as much as you can.

● Find out if your work is hazardous to pregnancy (see p. 33).
● Ask your doctor to check your immunity to German measles – rubella (see p. 24).

The blastocyst, now an embryo, consists of three layers from which all body structures will develop.

WEEKS 5–6

You may start to feel pregnant – changes in the breasts, feelings of nausea and your tastes may change. Frequency of urination. Urine test would give a positive result by now.

The baby's head is forming, the heart is beating and the legs are growing. The placenta is developing, though it is still not ready to take over from the ovary.

WEEKS 6–8

You should visit your doctor to confirm the pregnancy. Your doctor will give you a thorough physical examination. Have a preliminary discussion with your doctor about the possible type of birth (see Chapter 3) and the prenatal care you will have (Chapter 4). Use this visit to determine your doctor's views on labor and birth. Ask about pre-registration for a hospital birth.

All the baby's internal organs are in place. Nearly 1 in long.

Week 8

Fetal length
1 in

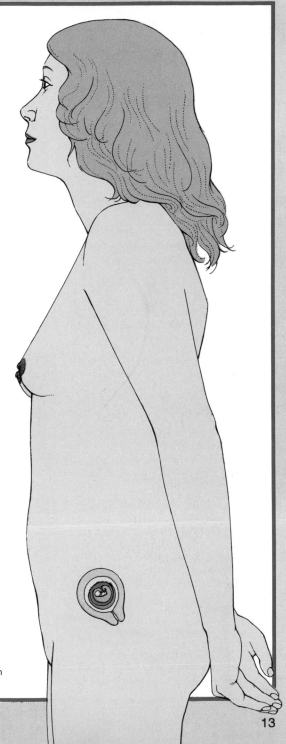

WEEK 10

May notice gain in weight if not before. Your breasts will be heavier – wear a good, supporting bra. Amount of blood in body increases steadily from now on. Heart and lungs begin to work harder. Kidneys increase their work; may cause a deficiency of necessary nutrients, so watch your diet. Keep up your normal fitness routine after first checking with your doctor. Book a dental appointment.

Tell your employer that you are expecting a baby and find out maternity benefits.

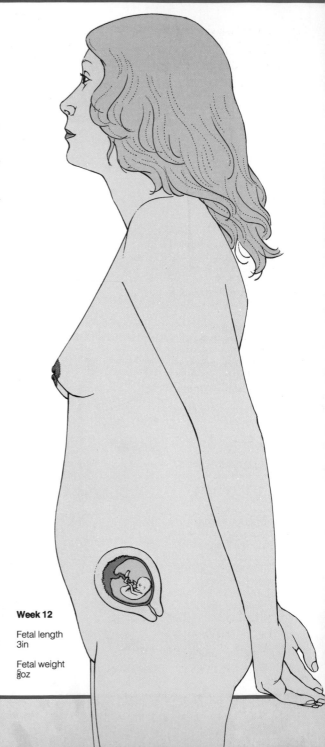

Baby is moving around a lot though you can't feel it. Eyes are well formed, fingers and toes develop, though they are joined by webs of skin.

WEEK 12

Nausea begins to diminish and frequency of urination eases. May experience constipation as the bowel slows down. By this week your uterus has risen above your pelvis. Baby's heartbeat can be heard with a Doppler probe by now.

- You will have your doctor's appointments now monthly until 28 weeks.
- Feel free to ask questions.
- If your doctor opts for ultrasound, you will be booked for an ultrasonic scan; check why first (see p. 66).

Week 12

Fetal length
3in

Fetal weight
$\frac{5}{8}$oz

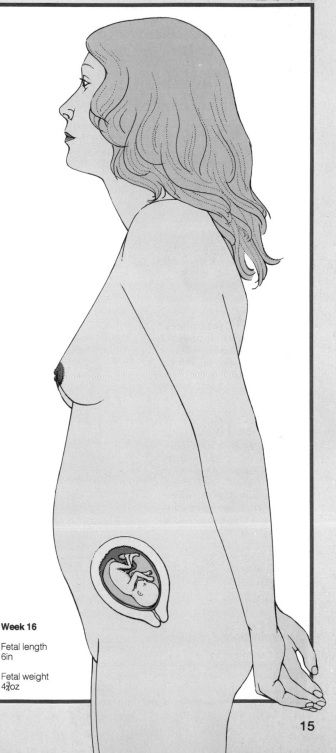

External genitals are clear. Face is properly formed and the muscles are developing so that the baby's movements are becoming stronger.

WEEK 14

Will start to feel better and more energetic. Nipples and areolas have noticeably darkened. If you haven't done so already, go out and buy a good bra with adequate support (see p. 83).

- Now that you feel better, you should plan your exercise program.
- Sign up for prenatal exercise classes.
- If you have had previous problems with an incompetent cervix, now is the time when the suture will be inserted under a general anesthetic (see p. 146).

Your baby is completely formed. From now on it grows in size rather than complexity and the formation of vital organs is unlikely to be harmed by drugs, infections or poisons. Increase in weight pronounced. Placenta has formed and is beginning to work.

WEEK 16

You will now probably be noticeably pregnant. Muscles and ligaments begin to slacken, your waistline disappears.

Week 16

Fetal length
6in

Fetal weight
4¾oz

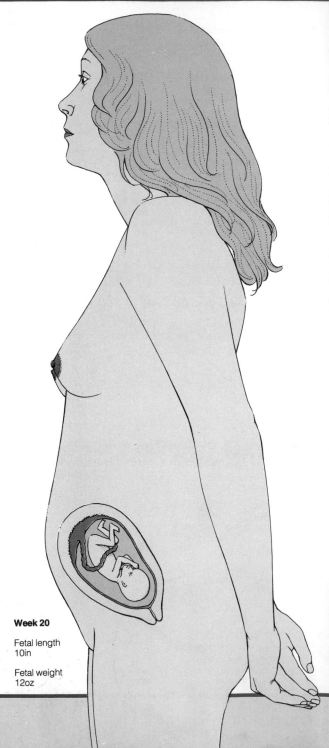

Start wearing comfortable, unrestricting clothes (see p. 122). Choose your food carefully; your appetite will increase and weight gain can be rapid. If your nipples invert, you could start to wear breast shields for an hour a day to get used to them (see p. 123).

● If indicated, amniocentesis will be performed (see p. 68). Results take about 3 weeks to come through.
● Ask your doctor about signing up for childbirth preparation classes, if you haven't already done so.

Baby is growing very fast in length and its movements may be vigorous. Fine hair appears all over its body (lanugo). Placenta is fully formed and functioning.

WEEK 18

Baby's movements can now be felt as light butterfly-like ripples. Results of your blood tests will show whether or not you are Rhesus negative (see p. 151).
Results of amniocentesis will be given to you soon.

Arms and legs are well formed and baby can twist and turn within the uterine sac.

WEEK 20

May notice increase in pigmentation, and if you want to, you can express colostrum in preparation (see p. 83).

Week 20

Fetal length
10in

Fetal weight
12oz

If chloasma appears on your face, avoid the sun and don't bleach it (see p. 126).

Baby's teeth start to form in the jawbone; hair appears on its head. If it's your first baby, you (and your partner) will definitely feel the baby's movements by now.

WEEK 24

Your most rapid weight gain takes place about now; your feet will start to feel the strain. Check that your shoes are right (see p. 124). Rest with your feet up whenever possible. By week 25 your heart and lungs are doing 50 per cent more work. You will generally sweat more because of raised body fluid levels. Ensure your salt intake is adequate. Keep up the exercising. You will look more flushed with the increase in blood circulation underneath the skin. Make the most of it. This is the best time in a pregnancy for many women.

The baby is still very thin but lengthening. It can suck its thumb and hiccup. Creases appear on its palms and fingertips.

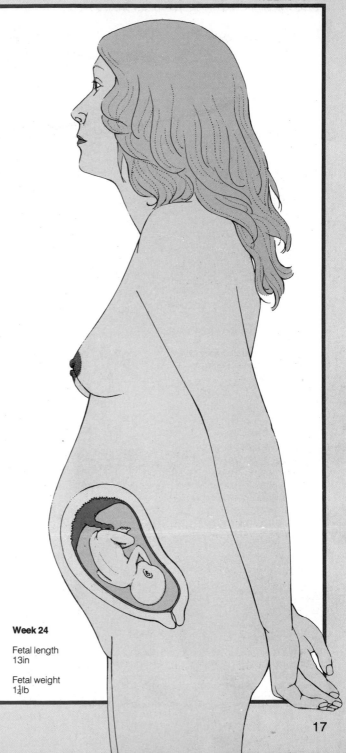

Week 24

Fetal length
13in

Fetal weight
1¼lb

17

WEEK 28

The skin on your abdomen becomes very stretched and thin and stretchmarks, if you have them, will be obvious. Your visit to the doctor will be every two weeks from now until 36 weeks. If your baby was born, it would have a good chance of survival. If indigestion is a problem, eat little and often and keep up your calcium intake with dairy products, particularly if you suffer with cramps. Some of the minor problems of pregnancy (see Chapter 12) will have become a part of your life. Approach any problems sensibly, and be assured they will disappear after the birth. You should be getting plenty of rest and sleep. Your childbirth preparation classes may start about now. You might want to find out whether infantcare classes are also available.

You should make your arrangements for maternity leave; talk to your employer to confirm plans.

Baby's head is now smaller in comparison with the body. Fat is beginning to accumulate and a fatty substance – vernix – coats the baby's skin so it doesn't get soggy in the amniotic fluid.

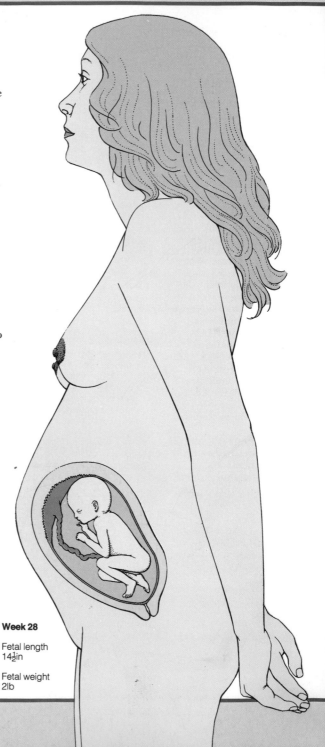

Week 28

Fetal length
14½in

Fetal weight
2lb

WEEK 32

You will be exhausted and perhaps breathless on exertion. You may have more blood tests. If your baby is in the breech position (bottom down), you may have external version to turn it head down (see p. 192). Movements can be clearly felt and seen on ultrasonic scans. As the uterus rises, you may suffer soreness on the lower edge of the ribcage as the baby and uterus push up under your diaphragm. Your navel will be flattened out and the linea nigra will be clearly seen running down your abdomen.

● If you can, slow down your schedule. Prepare a suitcase for a hospital birth or get in the necessary items for a home birth (see p. 156)
● Take things easy; especially if you aren't sleeping well. Rest as much as you can.

The baby is perfectly formed and in most cases will have turned head down (cephalic). If born now, it has a 50 per cent chance of survival because its lungs are developed. The placenta has reached maturity.

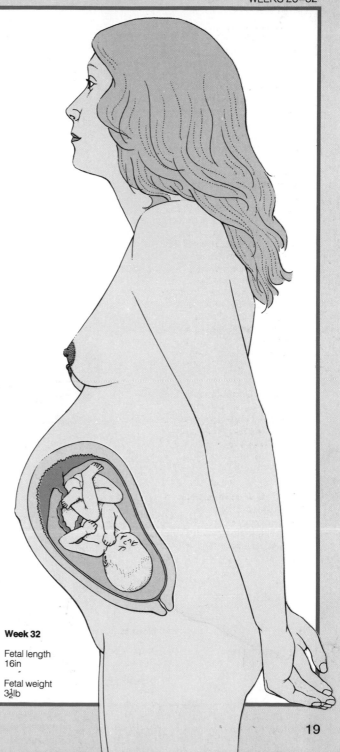

Week 32

Fetal length
16in

Fetal weight
3½lb

WEEK 36

Visits to the doctor will be weekly now until delivery. If this is your first baby, the head will engage (see p. 159). This will ease breathing problems but pain may be felt in the pelvic region. Urination increases again. Don't stand for too long; your ankles may swell. Rest with your feet up as much as possible. Plan your life carefully; don't organize too much activity, but keep yourself entertained with hobbies or books. The nesting instinct may become quite strong. Strong Braxton Hicks contractions may make you believe you are in labor. Practice your breathing techniques with the Braxton Hicks (see p. 163).

Buy good nursing bras if you plan to breastfeed. Your breasts won't enlarge until the milk comes in after the birth. You may need to wear breast pads if colostrum is secreted and any vaginal secretions could require light, stick-on sanitary pads (never internal tampons).

The baby is getting steadily plumper. Irises of the eyes are now blue. Fingernails reach to the ends of the fingers.

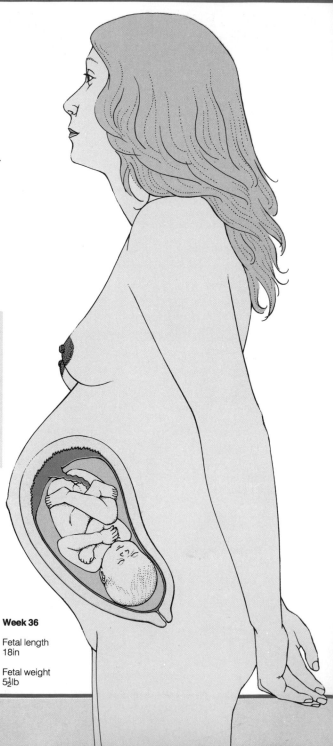

Week 36

Fetal length
18in

Fetal weight
5½lb

20

WEEK 40 (TERM)

With second and subsequent babies, the head engages. The expected date of delivery is near; you may become anxious when it passes, but only about 5 per cent of babies arrive on the due date. The baby's movements decrease as there is less space in the uterus, but strong jabs from hands and feet can still be felt.

The baby is about 20in long and weighs on average 7½lb. In a boy the testicles have descended.

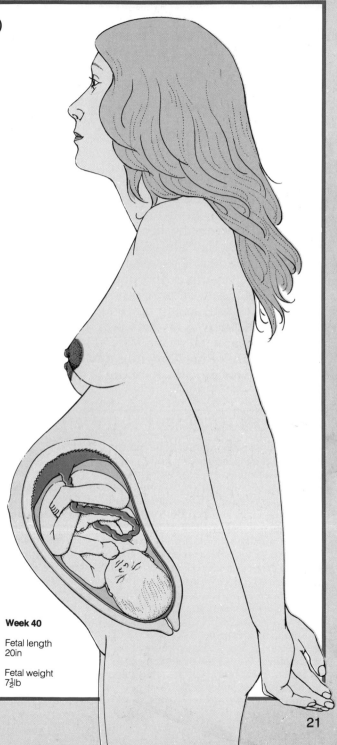

Week 40

Fetal length
20in

Fetal weight
7½lb

1 Deciding to have a baby

The professor of Obstetrics at my medical school used to tell us that there was no right time to have a baby because something else always came up in a couple's professional or domestic life. The corollary of this is that there is no wrong time to have a baby either. Paramount in the decision to have a baby, however, is that it is wanted. For many couples this means that the baby ideally should be planned. Even planning is often not as perfect as we would like nor, in my opinion, should it be. For one thing a woman may not find it easy to conceive once she has made the decision. Babies cannot be made to order.

After much soul-searching about interrupting my career I decided to have my first baby in my 35th year. I stopped the oral contraceptive pill and soon became pregnant. When I wanted my second child, however, I failed to conceive for 12 months and they were 12 months of anguish. So be prepared for the best planning to go awry.

ARE YOU HEALTHY ENOUGH?

Every year a small number of babies are born who are not as healthy as they might be. There are many reasons why this should happen. But far and away the two most important factors are the nutrition and fitness of the mother. Both of these things not only affect the health and well-being of your baby, but they also can help to determine whether you have a smooth or difficult pregnancy, labor and birth. It is important to pay close attention to diet and lifestyle as well as your general state of health *before* you make the decision to have a baby (see p. 101). Ideally you should also determine to get yourself fit before conception and keep yourself fit during the whole of the pregnancy and lactation. Your body will then be able to cope with the stresses and strains of pregnancy.

Diet

If you are not already doing so, you can improve your health enormously by paying attention to your diet. You may think you eat well, but look closely. Do you skip breakfast and eat a small lunch, saving your appetite for an evening meal? If you have children, do you leave the fresh fruit for them? Do you get so hungry during the day that you resort to cookies and high-calorie foods to get you through? You can improve your health almost immediately (see pp. 96–101) by increasing your intake of fresh fruit, vegetables and high-fiber foods and cutting down on highly refined, starchy foods and candy.

If you prepare for pregnancy, you will have less cause to worry about your health and the baby's.

Exercise

If you lead a sedentary life you should try to fit in some kind of exercise, either a sport such as tennis or swimming or an exercise program using a rowing machine or an exercise bicycle. Try to take some form of exercise every day for at least 20 minutes, during which time you should get slightly out of breath and sweat a bit. If this sounds daunting, start with a brisk walk, which is better than nothing.

Drugs

You should take particular care to cut down on the "social" drugs before you conceive – the major one being cigarettes (see p. 105). The risks of smoking are fully accepted, even the risks to those who do not smoke. This includes the people you live with. A woman living with people who smoke takes in a lot of nicotine and tars in the cigarette smoke in the air around her.

If you possibly can, you should try to give up smoking before conception; it may take you some time to kick the habit, so when you *decide* to have a baby, then is the time to stop smoking.

Smoking is associated with infertility in women, though the effects on male fertility may be more damaging. Sperm are more at risk than eggs, and it is believed that smoking could cause damage to the chromosomes in the cells of smokers.

For many years it was thought that the social drug marijuana had little effect on reproduction. In fact the latest tests show that it can interfere with the normal production of male sperm which, if united with an ovum, may result in an abnormal baby. Both parents owe it therefore to their baby to refrain from smoking marijuana for nine months before they decide to conceive. Other drugs should also be avoided (see p. 107).

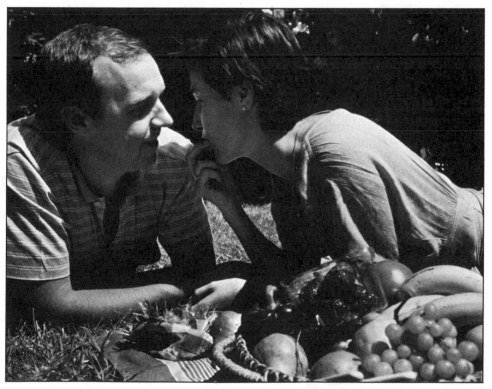

Alcohol is another social drug that can affect your pregnancy (see p. 106). It is increasingly being linked to certain birth defects and in severe cases to a syndrome producing physical and mental abnormalities.

Age of the parents

Age will always be a factor for you to consider when deciding to have a baby but not the negative one that you might think. More and more women are waiting until they are over 30 to become pregnant but many women fear that they may be waiting too long. This is because they have heard that the longer they wait the greater is the likelihood of having a difficult pregnancy or even, possibly, a defective child. The risk of having a Down's syndrome baby, for example, increases with maternal age (see p. 69). Carefully documented case studies, however, show that it is not dangerous for a woman to defer pregnancy until she is past her 20s and every older woman need not be considered a high risk.

The risks undoubtedly do increase with age, but every decision to have a child is unique and the age of the parents only one factor, and a very small one, in weighing up the risks and benefits. The age of the father relates more to infertility than to risk. Many other factors affect the risk factor ratio for the mother. One is the mother's socio-economic status. Of course, what these statistics do is to lump all mothers over the age of, say, 30 together, whether they are sick or well, rich or poor. The complications during pregnancy and delivery for this group are not related to age but to other factors such as malnutrition. In many cases an individual woman will need special care only if she is malnourished, regardless of her age.

Many experts have come up with the "best" age to have a baby, be it 18–20, 20–25, or 25–30. In most cases, however, women have no choice. When she is younger, a woman may be too involved with her career to have children or she may not have met the right person to be the father of her children. Many women simply are not ready to settle down until they are over 30. Though fertility does diminish with age (see p. 32), an important factor to consider is that the statistics show that the odds are greatly in favour of your having a successful pregnancy at almost any age. Many studies have been done on normal pregnancies in women past the age of 50 and all of them concluded that the general health of the mother is much more important than age alone as a factor in predicting how the pregnancy will turn out. So remember, if your health is good, the decision to have a baby should not be abandoned on account of age alone.

RUBELLA

Malformation, including deafness, blindness and heart disease, may occur if your developing baby is exposed to the virus of German measles (rubella), especially during the first three months when all the vital organs are forming and developing.

What to do

If you have not had German measles as a child or been vaccinated against it at puberty, consult your doctor and ask for a blood test to find out whether or not you are immune. If you are not immune, you should be vaccinated against rubella. You should then wait at least three months before trying to conceive. If you are already pregnant, your initial blood test will show if you have immunity. If you have not, and you come into contact with the disease, tell your doctor at once. Blood tests taken every two weeks will show if you have become infected. If you do become infected, you may have to make the difficult decision to terminate your pregnancy.

Pre-existing medical conditions

In some women, their general medical condition may make the pregnancy and labor difficult. However, with careful prenatal care and monitoring, and perhaps hospitalization in the last trimester, these women should have a normal birth. Conditions requiring special attention include diabetes, heart disease and RH blood incompatibility (see pp. 144–151). Women who are undertaking a long-term drug treatment, for epilepsy for example, should talk to their doctors about their treatment before conceiving.

EFFECTS ON LIFESTYLE

A recent survey showed that the number of women in America who consider motherhood the most pleasurable aspect of being a woman has dropped in the last ten years. Conversely, the number of women who feel that work is more fulfilling has risen. As women have examined their status in society more and more over the past decade and decided to be more self-determined than in the past, aided by reliable contraceptive methods, fewer are taking the role of wife and mother as the automatic choice in life. The investment of more time in the pursuit of a career also means that more women are opting to have families later in their lives. Both of these things have meant that the majority of women no longer have children and become mothers because of custom or by accident. The decision to be a mother and have children is more often than not a well-considered one. Most of us at any rate would condemn the unquestioned idealization of the act of childbearing that made society view it as essential to woman's fulfillment.

Some women, as they get older and fear that their fertility is diminishing, but have not found a partner they wish to settle down with, regard single parenthood as a possible choice. Women who make this decision and conceive a baby are usually remarkable for their single-mindedness and are quite prepared to face the problems. To them motherhood is a chosen state, not one that is imposed by chance.

Anxiety about parenthood

When you consider the change in lifestyle, the possible disruption of a happy relationship, the concessions and adjustments that have to be made with the advent of a baby, the choice of not having children at all becomes more understandable than it might have been. Many people, when they stop to think about it, fear parenthood. It's a reasonable anxiety: it is natural to worry about coping with the child's upbringing and worrying about your child's happiness if things go wrong. There will be economic pressures, the problem of resuming your career and possible frustration due to loss of freedom. As a couple you may have had two incomes to live on and your pregnancy may mean that for some time you are going to have to manage on one. Not everyone relishes the fact that they are no longer free agents; you are quite normal if you question your ability to feel loving and caring towards your baby all the time. In normal life you are beseiged by many negative feelings such as resentment, bitterness, irritation, bad temper, misanthropy, and there is no reason to think that the presence of your baby will call an end to these feelings.

It is perhaps only when you become a parent that you realize how much is demanded of you. In the early years your baby is an unscrupulous taker. But the one lesson that I have learned is that the more you give the more is given back to you as your child grows older.

Father's role

The role of the modern father has changed too. More and more commonly fathers take the responsibility for being a parent very seriously and are not prepared to be strangers to their children. For many years men were shut out of pregnancy and from the day-to-day care of their children on the assumption that it was woman's work and not their place. But liberated mothers have fostered liberated fathers. These fathers now feel free to indulge all their paternal instincts; they want to be involved with their partner during pregnancy and delivery; and they are not prepared to miss out on their children's growing up. The modern father is an active father rather than a passive one. Even in the early years your child will reward you with irreplaceable moments of pleasure, possibly pride, and as she grows older, more and more hours of companionship, love, comfort and joy.

Most fathers who have a keen interest in the pregnancy stay interested after the baby is born. Studies have shown that a father becomes more closely attached to his baby according to how much he holds it in the first six weeks of life and whether he answers the baby's cry. His attitude is also affected by his partner's enjoyment of pregnancy and motherhood. The happier a man is about his partner's pregnancy and the more he looks forward to enjoying

fatherhood, the more he will get out of the first few weeks of his baby's life.

Sharing responsibilities

Most couples agree that parents should be equal and that the roles of parenting and childraising must be equally shared. When you decide to have a baby you and your partner should view it as a contract: a contract which states that you are equally responsible for raising the child you have conceived. You should try to discuss and agree with each other on the roles that you want to play. A woman no longer expects to be the sole nursemaid, childminder and babysitter, confined to the house with its limited horizons and interests, while the father leaves home early and doesn't return until the baby is asleep. More and more women are unwilling partners in this kind of arrangement. These are some of the points that must be resolved between you before the baby is born if you want to provide a happy and stable environment in which to raise your child and be satisfied in your new role.

DISCONTINUING CONTRACEPTION

If you are taking the oral contraceptive pill, you should plan to have three normal menstrual periods before you become pregnant to allow your metabolic functions to return to normal after discontinuing the pill. During the intervening months you should use some mechanical form of contraception such as the condom or a cervical cap (see p. 223).

Much has been written about a woman's return to fertility after taking the pill, particularly if she has been taking it for long periods of time. When the pill first came into fashion it was thought that fertility was increased after its withdrawal as the body overcompensated for long periods of suppressed fertility. We now know that this is not necessarily so. Then there were scares about infertility following the pill, but large studies have shown that the majority of women

conceive in the first year after stopping the pill and nearly all women after two years.

If you suspect that you have become pregnant while taking the pill, you should consult your doctor immediately. There is a slight risk to the embryo from the hormones in the oral contraceptive pill during the very early phase of its development.

There is no need to put off conception after removing an I.U.D. However, if you become pregnant with an I.U.D. *in utero* it would be advisable to have it removed as soon as pregnancy is confirmed if you wish to continue the pregnancy. I.U.D.s left in place can result in spontaneous abortion, premature delivery and infection. Although doctors may tell you stories of delivering normal babies when an I.U.D. has been in the uterus for the whole of the pregnancy, this is not recommended.

GETTING PREGNANT

Knowing about your natural body cycles will give you enough information both to conceive and to avoid conception. The three body rhythms that you can observe are your monthly menstrual cycles, your daily body temperature and the appearance and consistency of the cervical mucus (your vaginal discharge).

Observing body rhythms

Most women have menstrual cycles of varying length. After recording your menstrual cycles, say for four months, if you find that the shortest one was 26 days and the longest one was 32 days, then using the following chart you can see that your fertile days are from the 9th to the

Record of menstrual cycle

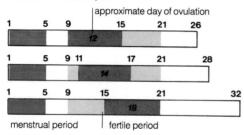

menstrual period | fertile period

21st day of each cycle. For conception, these are the days to concentrate on.

A woman's body temperature drops and then rises just before ovulation. Take your temperature each morning before you get

out of bed and chart it on a daily temperature chart (see below) for several months. A regular pattern will emerge and you will be able to see which day you ovulate after the onset of menstruation. You are fertile for one day before the temperature drops, while it remains elevated and for one day afterwards.

Your vaginal discharge goes through a cycle of changes as the month progresses. Just after menstruation there is hardly any discharge, but it is cloudy, sticky and thick. As you approach the fertile period it becomes abundant, clear and stretchy. As soon as you notice this change you have entered the few days when you can conceive. Fertility wanes when the discharge becomes cloudy, sticky and thick once again.

Frequency of intercourse

It is not true that conception is helped by frequent intercourse. In fact the opposite is true. The more often a man ejaculates the fewer sperm are contained in his ejaculate. The number may drop below the minimum required for conception. If you are trying to have a baby, it is a good idea for your partner to abstain from intercourse for a few days before your fertile period so that the numbers of sperm will rise. You should also have intercourse no more often than once daily during your fertile days.

Daily temperature chart

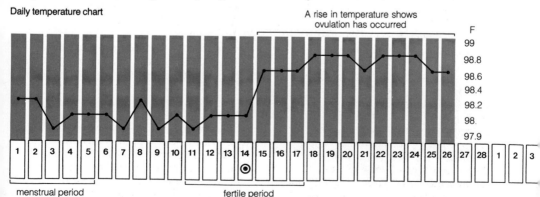

A rise in temperature shows ovulation has occurred

menstrual period | fertile period

27

INFLUENCE OF CHROMOSOMES AND GENES

Each cell in the body contains 46 chromosomes in 23 pairs, one half of each pair coming from the father's sperm and the other half from the mother's ovum. Each chromosome consists of a chain of about two thousand genes strung together. Genes carry the physical and intellectual characteristics that we derive directly from our parents. For example, characteristics such as the color of the eyes, or the curliness of the hair, have a gene from the mother and father. For each characteristic there is a dominant and recessive form. The gene for dark hair, for example, is always dominant over the gene for blond hair; likewise brown eyes will always dominate the gene for blue eyes. Nevertheless, both genes are present though one is masked. This is why two dark-haired parents can have a blond child in whom hair color is represented by the masked blond from the mother and the masked blond from the father.

One pair out of the 23 pairs of chromosomes determines a person's gender. Sperm cells are of two types – X, which are female, and Y, which are male. Ova only come in the X, or female form, so men have a sex chromosome of the XY type and women have the XX type. Biologically the male is responsible for the sex of the baby. If the Y sperm unites with the ovum, the baby will be a boy (XY) but if it's an X that unites with the ovum the baby will be a girl (XX). Scientists have discovered that the Y sperm has a longer tail, is produced in greater numbers, and moves faster than the female or X sperm, which has more staying power and therefore survives longer. If you wish to try for a boy or a girl, there are certain conditions that may favor conception with either the Y or the X sperm.

The masked gene for blond hair can occur with brown-haired parents with dazzling results.

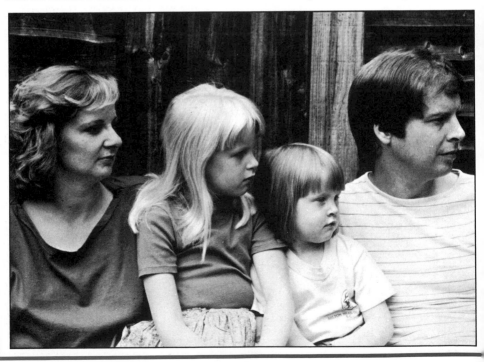

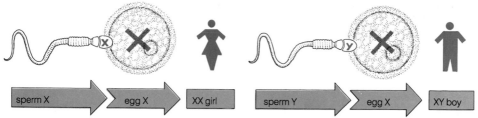

| sperm X | egg X | XX girl |

| sperm Y | egg X | XY boy |

Determining the child's sex
This occurs at the moment of conception. If the sperm carries an X chromosome, the baby will be a girl; if the sperm carries a Y chromosome, the baby will be a boy. The ovum carries only an X (female) chromosome.

To conceive a girl

● Stop intercourse two to three days before ovulation so that the male sperm will die, leaving only female sperm for fertilization.
● Have intercourse frequently to lower the numbers of male sperm.
● An acid environment favors female sperm, so douche the vagina with one part vinegar to ten parts water before you have intercourse.

To conceive a boy

● So that the faster male sperm reach the egg first, have intercourse on or as near to ovulation as possible.
● Have intercourse only once in 24 hours to increase the proportion of male sperm in the semen.
● To make the vagina more favorable to male sperm, douche with a solution of one teaspoon of bicarbonate of soda to 1 pint water.

Genetic counselling

Quite rightly emphasis is put on the mother's health because it is crucial to give the baby a healthy environment in which to develop. But the health of the father is crucial, too. Large numbers of normal sperm give the best possible chance for a healthy union between the egg and his sperm; only in healthy men is there the healthy production of sperm. If the father's sperm or the mother's egg are greatly defective, they may not be able to unite at all to form an embryo. If they are only slightly defective, it is possible for a baby to develop that is not quite normal. Every year 150,000 children are born in the United States with congenital malformations. The majority of these cannot be anticipated and occur purely because of random selection. If with either partner, however, there is a history of a disease or condition which runs through family members and generations, then you should seek genetic counselling. These conditions include hemophilia and Down's syndrome. Having a baby is by no means precluded, but your decision to go ahead and try can only be helped by having specialized information. A chromosome count may be able to give you some idea as to what the risks are of having an abnormal child. In this simple, painless procedure, some cells are gently scraped from the inside of your mouth and are then examined under a microscope.

All of us take some risk, albeit a minute one, when we decide to have a baby. Knowing how your risk compares to everyone else's is information that you cannot do without. If it's a small one you may decide to go ahead and try. If, however, the risk is very great, you may decide that you would prefer to adopt a child.

FERTILIZATION

As a general rule fertilization happens about a week after you have finished menstruating or 14 days before your next menstrual period. About 7 to 10 days after this the fertilized ovum becomes implanted in the lining of the womb. By the end of another week it is firmly attached by its primitive placenta, which links the developing embryo to its mother (see p. 71). The placenta is the organ through which nutrients are carried from the mother to the baby and waste substances from the baby to the mother. It is an absolutely crucial organ to the healthy progress of pregnancy because it produces pregnancy hormones that are responsible for maintaining the health of the developing baby, the uterus and the female genital organs and preparing the woman's body for the labor and birth.

The ovum is fertilized about a third of the way along the Fallopian tube by a sperm deposited in the vagina after ejaculation. Within a few seconds of ejaculation the sperm, which are invisible to the naked eye, become mobile, lashing their whiplike tails. This can carry them at top speed out of the acid conditions of the vagina and through the neck of the cervix, which during ovulation becomes thinner and invites entry, into the cavity of the uterus. In a few seconds the sperm crosses

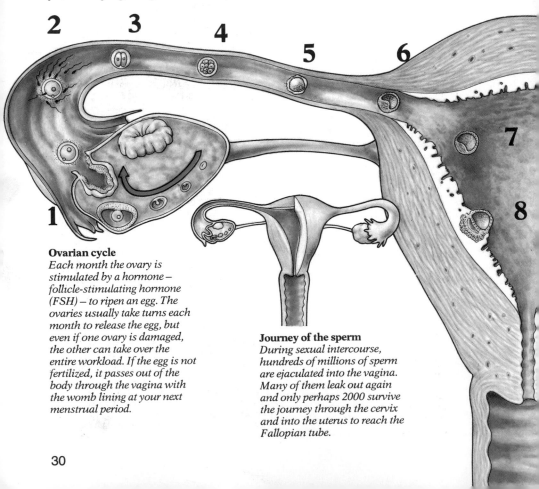

Ovarian cycle
Each month the ovary is stimulated by a hormone – follicle-stimulating hormone (FSH) – to ripen an egg. The ovaries usually take turns each month to release the egg, but even if one ovary is damaged, the other can take over the entire workload. If the egg is not fertilized, it passes out of the body through the vagina with the womb lining at your next menstrual period.

Journey of the sperm
During sexual intercourse, hundreds of millions of sperm are ejaculated into the vagina. Many of them leak out again and only perhaps 2000 survive the journey through the cervix and into the uterus to reach the Fallopian tube.

the uterus and enters the Fallopian tube. Sperm are chemically attracted to the comparatively enormous ovum and attach themselves like limpets over the whole surface. However, only one sperm pierces the outer coat of the ovum. Instantly the egg loses its attraction, hardens its outer shell and all the superfluous sperm let go. This whole process of ejaculation to fertilization usually takes less than 60 minutes.

The ripe ovum can probably survive for only 12 hours, a maximum of 24. Sperm retain the power to fertilize for about 24–48 hours. Fertilization is therefore unlikely unless sexual intercourse occurs one or two days before or immediately after ovulation.

Only the head of the sperm fuses with the ovum to form a single cell. The body and tail are lost. The cell divides into two in the first 24 hours and by the fourth day is a round ball made up of over 100 cells. For the first three days in the cavity of the uterus this ball of cells floats free, being nurtured on uterine "milk" secreted by the glands of the uterine wall. At the end of the first week of life it has burrowed deep into the lining – this is called implantation – where it is continuously bathed in a lake of its mother's blood, which facilitates the passage of food and waste to and from the embryo. Until week 8 of your pregnancy the developing baby is known as an embryo. After this time it is called a fetus, which means "young one" in Latin.

1 *The ovum is liberated from the surface of the ovary around the 14th day of the cycle. It is caught in the funnel-shaped end of the Fallopian tube and is propelled along it by muscular contractions.*

2 *Fertilization by one sperm usually occurs about a third of the way along the tube.*

3 *The fertilized cell divides in two within 24 hours.*

4 *With repeated cell divisions a ball of cells is formed.*

5 *The egg continues to divide as it is swept along the tube.*

6 *A hollow cavity, known as the blastocyst, forms in the ball of cells.*

7 *The blastocyst reaches the cavity of the uterus.*

8 *Implantation begins around day 7 and is most commonly in the upper part of the uterus on either side depending on whether the left or right ovary ovulated. By day 10 the embryo is firmly embedded.*

CONCEPTION OF TWINS
If the egg released from the ovary is fertilized and then divides in two, identical twins with the same sex result, sharing the same placenta. More commonly (in 70 per cent of twins) two eggs may be fertilized by two sperm. These fraternal twins have separate placentas and amniotic sacs.

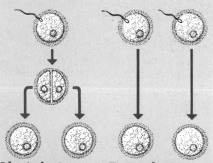

Identical twins
The egg is fertilized and then splits into separate cells. This split can even occur after the egg is implanted in the uterus.

Fraternal twins
In the majority of twins two eggs are released into the Fallopian tube and then two sperm fertilize them independently.

INFERTILITY

About one in every ten women of childbearing age is subfertile and unable to have babies. This ratio is fairly constant throughout the Western nations. Infertility, however, is not a matter of either partner exclusively but of the couple as a unit. Your fertility is indivisible from the fertility of you and your partner together. In some circumstances the high fertility of one partner can compensate for the low fertility of the other. On the other hand, marginal fertility in both partners may result in sterility. This would explain the paradox of a childless couple splitting up and then both partners producing children without any difficulty in a new partnership.

Female infertility

In women one of the most important factors that affects fertility is age. Fertility begins to diminish around the age of 25 (see below). After the age of 45 only half a woman's cycles are ovulatory, so she has only half as many fertile periods during the year as a younger woman. Her fertility is consequently much reduced. The decline in a man's fertility is more gradual. It is the same as a woman's at the age of 20 and wanes slowly to 10 per cent by the age of 60.

In many women the desire for children can be intense and overriding. Many women become physically ill with the desire to conceive. I well understand and

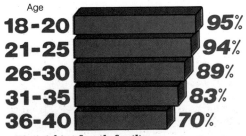

Age

18-20	95%
21-25	94%
26-30	89%
31-35	83%
36-40	70%

Diminishing female fertility
The reduction in fertility is only slight until 35, when conception becomes more difficult and the risks of pregnancy are increased (see p. 64).

sympathize with this uncontrollable desire. I myself was infertile – in a sense – between the birth of my first and second baby. Each month I observed my body for signs of menstruation and was hysterical with grief when the period came. I was just as obsessed, just as depressed as any woman who cannot have children at all. It was only at the end of the year when I forced myself to be more philosophical that conception occurred.

The barriers to fertility can be physical, psychological and emotional. Many people find the subject difficult and too embarrassing to discuss, but if as a couple you wish to have your subfertility investigated, you will need to seek help from a doctor, a marriage counselor or a psychiatrist. That means both of you discussing sensitive subjects in an open and sensible way.

Examining a woman's infertility can involve the following procedures:
● keeping daily records of her menstrual cycle to see if she has ovulated
● examining vaginal secretions to see if they respond to hormone treatment
● surgical exploration, usually laproscopy, in which a telescope-like instrument is passed through the abdominal wall so that doctors can look at the condition of the genital tract
● passing a dye through your Fallopian tubes which is visible on an X-ray – this will show up any blockages
● taking blood or urine samples to estimate progesterone levels.
It's a time-consuming, lengthy and frustrating process, so you have to be psychologically prepared to carry it out. The failure to ovulate or produce sufficient numbers of sperm is amenable to stimulation by drugs. The same chemicals can be used by both men and women, though the results are much better in women. First a fairly simple drug is used in gradually increasing doses to stimulate ovulation until it occurs regularly. If this initial treatment fails, hormone therapy

may be considered. Pregnancy results in about two-thirds of patients who receive this form of therapy and usually within a short time, about three to four months. With careful dosage adjustment, multiple pregnancies are becoming rarer. However, miscarriages at the rate of approximately one in eight may occur in these induced pregnancies.

Male infertility

In men there are two main causes of infertility: a blockage in the tubes between the testes and the penis, and inadequate production of sperm. Before these problems can be excluded as possible causes of infertility, hospital investigation and laboratory tests will be required. Inadequate sperm production involves three kinds of deficiency: a low sperm count, low sperm mobility or large numbers of abnormal sperm. These characteristics have to be examined not only in the laboratory but in the woman after intercourse.

Artificial insemination

If the husband is impotent, then artificial insemination with his own sperm should result in pregnancy. This is known as AIH. If, however, the cause of infertility is too few sperm or too many abnormal sperm, then it's necessary to use the sperm of a donor, AID. This step should be undertaken only after careful consultation with your doctor. Some doctors, however, regard AID as an ethical question and they are entitled to refuse to co-operate. Where there is no impediment to conception in the wife, four out of every five women can expect to conceive within six months.

Women who have successfully used AID would argue in favor of it because they wish to bear their own child rather than adopting. Some couples even view AID as a kind of adoption, but with more similarities between themselves and their child than with a fully adopted child. There is a very low divorce rate in couples who use AID, which answers one of the questions raised by opponents who fear

that the child may be brought up in an unstable home. Some counter-arguments against AID include social concern about its effects on the family as well as religious concern about its moral acceptability. The important social concerns remain those involving the legal uncertainties about legitimacy, the child's status and the culpability of the wife if she uses AID without the consent of her husband.

HAZARDS AT WORK
If you or your partner work with certain chemicals, lead or radiation, your fertility could be affected. It is now known that certain industrial substances can damage sperm and cause malformed babies and spontaneous abortion. If you are not sure about the chemicals you work with and how they might affect your chances of conception, ask your doctor, union representative or personnel manager. If you can't avoid some contact with doubtful industrial substances, follow stringent safety regulations and wear protective clothing, avoid breathing in dust or fumes and avoid skin contact. Only a small number of the many substances used in industry have been recognized as needing a safety threshold. However, this safe level of exposure does not take into account how the chemicals affect fertility. Rather than taking a chance, if one of you works with a hazardous substance, you might like to change to a safer job before you conceive your baby.

If you are already pregnant, it may be dangerous for you to continue in a hazardous job – your baby could be at risk. Ask to be transferred to a safer job during your pregnancy. Check on your rights though: you could be dismissed fairly if there are no "safe" jobs for pregnant women in your industry or you are no longer able to do the job properly.

2 Finding out you are pregnant

There are two quite separate aspects to finding out you're pregnant. The first is a physical confirmation of your pregnancy that can be picked up in signs from your body like a feeling of nausea, having to empty your bladder more often and dilated veins on the surface of your breasts. Intellectual and emotional acceptance of your pregnancy is a quite different aspect. The first may be tinged with excitement and anxiety; the second for most of us is colored by feelings of ambivalence. No matter how much we've wanted to be pregnant, we nearly all have a mixed response to the news that we are.

A mixture of positive and negative feelings about the pregnancy is normal and nothing you should feel guilty about. Uppermost in your mind will be your feelings about yourself, your partner and your relationship. Many couples find they reassess each other before accepting their changing status. Eventually you will see that becoming parents can be a great step forward in your lives that introduces you to a thrilling and satisfying new role.

EARLY SYMPTOMS OF PREGNANCY

Perhaps the earliest sign of pregnancy is the feeling that you really are pregnant. There may have been times previously when you suspected that you were pregnant, but I think every woman knows when she really is. This feeling is not just to do with suspicions; there is a definite consciousness of being pregnant. I believe it has much to do with the first secretion of pregnancy hormones as anything else. The hormones affect your body in every respect, including your mind and the way you feel.

Another early sign is tiredness. Although some women feel energized, the majority, if asked, would confess to feeling tired. It is a new kind of tiredness that they haven't felt before. Some women say that they find themselves dropping off to sleep at any time of the day, sometimes within a few hours of getting up; others say that they become so sleepy in the early afternoon that they have to stop what they are doing for a few minutes and wait for the tiredness to pass. Others have pronounced fatigue in the evening. This tiredness, whenever it occurs, is often uncontrollable, and you may find that you just have to sleep. I have never found an explanation for this eccentric desire to sleep, but I feel it is an effect of progesterone, which reaches high levels in the blood early in pregnancy. Progesterone is a sedative in human beings (it's an anesthetic in horses) that has powerful tranquilizing and hypnotic effects.

Progesterone also accounts for the serene and beatific look that is classically associated with pregnancy. There is another type of fatigue occurring later in pregnancy (see p. 142), which is due simply to tiredness of the body, but it rarely occurs in the first trimester of pregnancy unless you are over-exerting yourself.

Missed period (amenorrhoea)

Within two weeks of fertilization you'll miss a period—the classic sign of pregnancy. While pregnancy is the commonest cause of amenorrhoea, it's not the only one, so don't automatically assume you're pregnant. A severe physical illness, a great shock, jet lag, even a surgical operation or anxiety are known to make a period late. On the other hand, it is quite common to have a very light period after the pregnancy is established; and this accounts for some pregnancies appearing to be only eight months in length (see p. 81).

Morning sickness

Many women suffer from sickness in one form or another, caused by the increasing levels of hormones circulating in the blood. One hormone called human hormone chorionic gonadotrophin (HCG) helps to maintain the pregnancy by keeping up supplies of estrogen and progesterone, thus preventing a menstrual period. It is the presence of HCG in urine that confirms a pregnancy (see p. 36). The build-up of this hormone roughly parallels the time of nausea for many women, tailing off at 12–14 weeks.

The sudden rush of hormones can have a direct irritant effect on the lining of the stomach, causing a feeling of nausea. Hormones also cause a rapid clearing of sugar from the blood, which can result in a feeling of great hunger and sickness. Nausea, in some cases accompanied by vomiting, occurs from about week 6. It rarely lasts longer than the first three months and then it gradually stops (see p. 138).

Tastes and cravings

A change in taste and in preferences for certain foods may be one of the first signs of pregnancy, occurring even before you miss a period. It is quite common to develop dislikes for certain foods and drink, commonly fried foods, coffee and alcohol, as well as cigarette smoke. It is often described as a metallic taste in the mouth which affects your appreciation of the food. Cravings are thought to be due to the rising hormone levels and are sometimes experienced during the second half of the menstrual cycle for the same reason. Don't indulge a craving for high-calorie foods, which may be low in nutritional value.

Frequency of urination (micturition)

As the uterus begins to swell, it presses on the bladder, which lies close to it. Consequently, the bladder tries to expel even small amounts of urine. Many women notice a desire to pass urine more frequently as early as one week after conception – you may find yourself having to go to the lavatory every hour. Unless there is a burning sensation or pain when you pass urine, there is no need to consult your doctor about increased frequency. By about week 12, the uterus has increased in size and rises up out of the pelvic cavity. This reduces the pressure on the bladder and the frequency for you.

Breasts

The changes that take place in the breasts in early pregnancy (see p. 82) are really an exaggerated form of what happens in the second half of every menstrual cycle due to stimulation by progesterone. Even before you miss your first period you will notice tingling and soreness of the nipples and your breasts may feel heavy and tender and be measurably larger. Very early in pregnancy the veins over the surface of the breasts become more prominent, and the creamy nodules in the nipple area become bigger. The nipples also start to enlarge and deepen in color. Your body is already preparing itself to nurture the baby.

RECEIVING THE NEWS

Most of us feel some ambivalence about being pregnant and find that our feelings shift with our moods. It's absolutely normal to have mixed feelings about pregnancy and parenthood. It would be unrealistic to imagine that your life will remain unchanged after the baby comes, so it's better to think ahead. Don't feel that you're inadequate for having conflicting

feelings and don't try to suppress them. It's far more sensible to acknowledge and face up to them, rather than trying to reach a point where there are no conflicts. This would be unrealistic.

Going through pregnancy is a phase of your emotional growth, and at the end of it you should have a better understanding and awareness of yourself.

PREGNANCY TESTS

Detecting the presence of the pregnancy hormone human chorionic gonadotrophin (see p. 82) in urine is the most common test. For it to be reliable, you must wait until two weeks after the first day of your missed period.

Home kits
These use a urine sample. Follow the manufacturer's instructions carefully as home kits vary. In the kit illustrated here, you add the chemical to the test tube and shake. Using the now empty tube, draw up some urine and add one drop to the chemical. Wait one hour. If the reflection forms a ring, the test is positive; if there is no pattern, the pregnancy test is negative.

Urine test
Pass a sample of your first urine of the morning into a clean, soap-free container. Your doctor will arrange for the test to be done. A negative result of a urine test does not necessarily mean you are not pregnant. If the other signs persist, try again in seven days; you may have tested too early in your pregnancy. Home kits and laboratory urine tests are 95 per cent reliable.

Internal examination
The doctor will insert two fingers into the vagina and by palpating your abdomen with the other hand, he or she can detect the general softening of the genital organs and the increase in size of the uterus. The test doesn't harm the embryo and is not reliable before the eighth week. The test is then 100 per cent reliable.

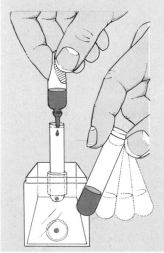

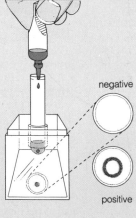

negative

positive

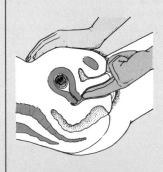

I am against the use of high-dose hormone tablets to test for pregnancy. If you are pregnant, the embryo could be affected.

Different reactions

The reactions to the confirmation of your pregnancy may not be what you expected them to be. It's possible that personal circumstances are such that a pregnancy is unwelcome. A woman may resent a pregnancy taking over and ruling her body; she may become bitter because her active life is curtailed. Some women become depressed when they realize they are pregnant and even consider abortion.

This is painting a negative picture, more negative perhaps than the majority of women feel. However, the most important part of receiving the news that you're pregnant is for you and your partner to accept the pregnancy fully. Don't think that you can ignore it and carry on as normal just because it doesn't show for the first few weeks or months. You both have to think of your pregnancy realistically, not in a rosy glow.

How to calculate your estimated date of confinement (EDC)

The average pregnancy is 266 days long from conception or 280 days measured from the first day of your last menstrual period (LMP). To find your EDC, find the date of your LMP in the columns of dates set in bold type, the date next to it is your EDC. You can also work it out as follows:

LMP   9.17.83
+ 9 months   6.17.84
+ 7 days   6.24.84

Remember 280 days is average and you may not be average. The possibility of your baby arriving on your EDC depends on your having regular 28-day cycles. All that doctors are prepared to say is that a normal pregnancy may be anywhere between 38 and 42 weeks.

Jan/Oct		Feb/Nov		Mar/Dec		Apr/Jan		May/Feb		June/Mar		July/Apr		Aug/May		Sept/June		Oct/July		Nov/Aug		Dec/Sept	
1	8	1	8	1	6	1	6	1	5	1	8	1	7	1	8	1	8	1	8	1	8	1	7
2	9	2	9	2	7	2	7	2	6	2	9	2	8	2	9	2	9	2	9	2	9	2	8
3	10	3	10	3	8	3	8	3	7	3	10	3	9	3	10	3	10	3	10	3	10	3	9
4	11	4	11	4	9	4	9	4	8	4	11	4	10	4	11	4	11	4	11	4	11	4	10
5	12	5	12	5	10	5	10	5	9	5	12	5	11	5	12	5	12	5	12	5	12	5	11
6	13	6	13	6	11	6	11	6	10	6	13	6	12	6	13	6	13	6	13	6	13	6	12
7	14	7	14	7	12	7	12	7	11	7	14	7	13	7	14	7	14	7	14	7	14	7	13
8	15	8	15	8	13	8	13	8	12	8	15	8	14	8	15	8	15	8	15	8	15	8	14
9	16	9	16	9	14	9	14	9	13	9	16	9	15	9	16	9	16	9	16	9	16	9	15
10	17	10	17	10	15	10	15	10	14	10	17	10	16	10	17	10	17	10	17	10	17	10	16
11	18	11	18	11	16	11	16	11	15	11	18	11	17	11	18	11	18	11	18	11	18	11	17
12	19	12	19	12	17	12	17	12	16	12	19	12	18	12	19	12	19	12	19	12	19	12	18
13	20	13	20	13	18	13	18	13	17	13	20	13	19	13	20	13	20	13	20	13	20	13	19
14	21	14	21	14	19	14	19	14	18	14	21	14	20	14	21	14	21	14	21	14	21	14	20
15	22	15	22	15	20	15	20	15	19	15	22	15	21	15	22	15	22	15	22	15	22	15	21
16	23	16	23	16	21	16	21	16	20	16	23	16	22	16	23	16	23	16	23	16	23	16	22
17	24	17	24	17	22	17	22	17	21	17	24	17	23	17	24	17	24	17	24	17	24	17	23
18	25	18	25	18	23	18	23	18	22	18	25	18	24	18	25	18	25	18	25	18	25	18	24
19	26	19	26	19	24	19	24	19	23	19	26	19	25	19	26	19	26	19	26	19	26	19	25
20	27	20	27	20	25	20	25	20	24	20	27	20	26	20	27	20	27	20	27	20	27	20	26
21	28	21	28	21	26	21	26	21	25	21	28	21	27	21	28	21	28	21	28	21	28	21	27
22	29	22	29	22	27	22	27	22	26	22	29	22	28	22	29	22	29	22	29	22	29	22	28
23	30	23	30	23	28	23	28	23	27	23	30	23	29	23	30	23	30	23	30	23	30	23	29
24	31	24	1	24	29	24	29	24	28	24	31	24	30	24	31	24	1	24	31	24	31	24	30
25	1	25	2	25	30	25	30	25	1	25	1	25	1	25	1	25	2	25	1	25	1	25	1
26	2	26	3	26	31	26	31	26	2	26	2	26	2	26	2	26	3	26	2	26	2	26	2
27	3	27	4	27	1	27	1	27	3	27	3	27	3	27	3	27	4	27	3	27	3	27	3
28	4	28	5	28	2	28	2	28	4	28	4	28	4	28	4	28	5	28	4	28	4	28	4
29	5			29	3	29	3	29	5	29	5	29	5	29	5	29	6	29	5	29	5	29	5
30	6			30	4	30	4	30	6	30	6	30	6	30	6	30	7	30	6	30	6	30	6
31	7			31	5			31	7			31	7	31	7			31	7			31	7

THE WORKING WOMAN

You will want to check the disability, insurance, and fringe benefit policies of your employer as soon as you know you are pregnant—or better yet, before you decide to conceive. If your employer has a disability policy, it applies to pregnancy as well as to illnesses or injuries. But if your employer has no disability policy, your pregnancy may not be covered at all. Find out, too, what company policy is concerning maternity leave. By law, you cannot be fired or refused promotion just because you are pregnant and the majority of employers will co-operate with plans that you may want to make for discontinuing your employment before the birth and for resuming it afterwards. You can expect no employer, however, to react

Whatever work you do, you'll find that your workmates are interested in your condition.

reasonably if you give little or no warning about your intentions. Around the end of the first trimester you should be thinking about your future work. Once you have discussed all your options and come to a decision, talk to your employer to see how your plans can be accommodated.

Working during pregnancy

Unless your work involves heavy physical labor, or you work in an environment where there are harmful chemicals or fumes (see p. 33), there is no reason why you should not continue working well into your pregnancy. The length of time that you will work depends on your physical fitness, the sort of job you are doing and your reasons for working. A psychological benefit of working that should not be overlooked is that it encourages everyone around you to view pregnancy as normal.

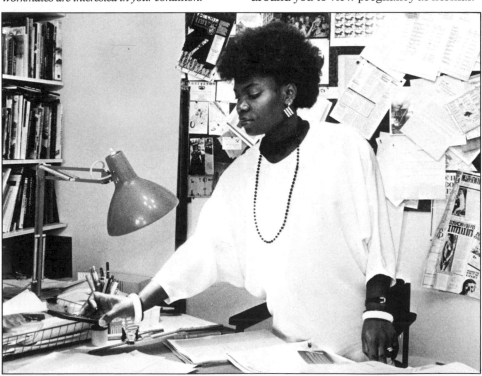

As well as that, your job gives you a feeling of stability and security during a time when you are undergoing physical and psychological changes.

Most medical authorities believe that if you have an uncomplicated pregnancy you can continue to work even up to the time of labor. At around 32 weeks, the greatest work load is thrown on your heart, lungs and other vital organs like the kidneys and liver, and there is a great deal of physical stress on your spine, your joints and muscles. It is a time when you should not be asking your body to do too much if you feel tired, except rest.

Whatever your job, you will have to make adjustments to your daily routine. As pregnancy progresses, you will lose some of your agility, and working long hours and having late nights will just leave you exhausted. You will find yourself falling asleep and losing concentration. As far as household chores are concerned, try to take a different attitude to them. Let your priorities slide. Your health and the health of your unborn child are more important.

TIPS FOR THE WORKING DAY

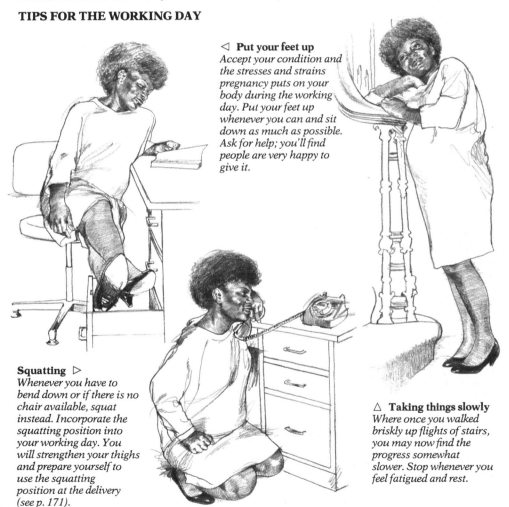

◁ **Put your feet up**
Accept your condition and the stresses and strains pregnancy puts on your body during the working day. Put your feet up whenever you can and sit down as much as possible. Ask for help; you'll find people are very happy to give it.

Squatting ▷
Whenever you have to bend down or if there is no chair available, squat instead. Incorporate the squatting position into your working day. You will strengthen your thighs and prepare yourself to use the squatting position at the delivery (see p. 171).

△ **Taking things slowly**
Where once you walked briskly up flights of stairs, you may now find the progress somewhat slower. Stop whenever you feel fatigued and rest.

Being a working mother

Some women are happy to deal with pregnancy as an interruption to their work, remaining in their posts until just before going into labor, having the baby and returning within a short time. They avoid the emotional dilemma of whether or not to breast or bottle feed the baby and opt for the latter. Other mothers, however, would be unhappy with this. They want to stay with and look after their children. Anything that takes them away from their children is painful. Women with strong maternal instincts will be concerned with not only depriving their babies of affection, but also with the sacrifices they are making themselves. These women crave the presence and company of their children, not all, but much of the time; especially when children are young it can be distressing to leave them even for a few hours a day.

Mothers nonetheless continue to work for many reasons, from economic necessity, from the desire to be independent and self-reliant, from boredom with the family and home, and from the absolute personal need to work. As women become freer to shape their own lives, more and more mothers are working and more and more simply because they enjoy it. They feel that work enriches their lives and if it does, that will certainly enrich family life. Until a decade or so ago, many women thought it was their duty to ignore their own desires and serve the family; now they feel very strongly that they have the right to take their own wishes into consideration and to make the decision to work, even knowing that it will create difficulties in the family.

The feelings of your partner should also be considered along with your own. It can lead only to unhappiness and resentment if you decide to return to work and your partner is reluctant for you to do so. If you have reason to believe that he feels this way, you must bring matters out into the open; a frank discussion with him may lead to a suitable compromise and a happy solution of your working future.

When to return

If you decide that you are going to return to work after your baby is born, you might want to return under different conditions. Discuss this with your employer. There may be provision for part-time employment in your work or a phased return which allows you to be in effect a part-time worker up until one year after the baby's birth. You might like to investigate job-sharing or going on your own in some freelance activity, which might enable you to work from home. Now is the time to think about these alternatives and plan for them.

In figuring out when you are going to restart work, you must be fair to yourself. It takes about nine months for your metabolism to return to normal after a pregnancy; parts of your body recover more quickly than others. If you menstruate three months after giving birth, this is a good sign that your ovaries are getting back to their normal cyclical routine, but not all your hormone glands will be in step with them. The muscles, ligaments and joints become more flexible and elastic to accommodate your pregnant shape and weight and need to regain their tone and strength. Vital organs like the heart, kidneys and lungs, and your blood, gradually adjust to coping with you alone and not with you plus the baby.

Babies and parents

A good system of childcare will be a priority; you'll have to put quite a lot of time and effort into selecting one that suits your needs. If you feel reluctant or guilty about entrusting your baby to someone else, fearing that you might be left out of your child's affections, be reassured as I was (even though only in retrospect) by an interesting study carried out in the last few years. When I actually was a working mother with small babies, I didn't know that this research was going on and trusted my own instinct. What I felt was that my children would know me as their mother by instinct, by the biological semaphore that I sent out and they picked

ADVANTAGES AND DISADVANTAGES OF BEING A WORKING MOTHER

Advantages

- increased independence
- financial rewards – chance to raise the standard of living of your family
- career fulfillment – chance to use whatever training and qualifications you may have
- more intense interaction with your child when you are at home
- intellectual fulfillment – bored and lonely at home
- need to maintain a high profile in your chosen field.

Disadvantages

- sense of guilt and inadequacy because you feel you are neglecting your child
- isolation from the community
- tiredness
- great stress due to the dual responsibilities and the need to be constantly planning ahead
- resentment of full-time mothers in your community
- worries about finding and keeping good childcare.

up. I felt certain in my own mind, despite the presence of very loving babysitters, that my children could never mistake a babysitter for me, their mother. When I thought about this I found it difficult to pin down how they would make the distinction. I thought possibly on body smell, and until they were about 18 months I made sure that they felt and smelt my skin at feeding times and during nuzzling play.

What research showed was that babies have an even keener intelligence for singling out their parents from all other human beings than I thought. The crucial factor isn't sight, smell or even physical contact, but the loving, interested attention that only parents can give, and that a baby sorts out from all other stimuli. The most staggering aspect of this research was the short length of time to which a baby has to be exposed to caring parental interest. Babies thrive with less than an hour a day. The length of time spent without their mother counts far less than the quality of the time spent with her. Love isn't measured in time, love is what you put into time, no matter how short.

Dual role

One of the aspects of being a working mother that makes life very hard is the necessity to invest all your free time in your family. You are working at two jobs;

there's no other way to look at it. Sometimes this is not too difficult. If, for instance, you have an intellectually taxing job, you may have the physical energy to spare when you get home for bathtimes, play, story reading and sympathetic listening. If, however, you are a teacher or a nurse, much of the sort of attention your children require will have been expended during your working day. Then it's doubly hard and there's no escape.

I firmly believe that a child, especially of pre-school age, has the right to expect and receive his parents' attention when they are home from work. The price of this is high. Instead of dropping into a chair when you return home, you'll have to pick up the baby and do everything else one-handed until he's asleep. Instead of climbing into a tub to soothe your shattered nerves, you'll have to cope with the bathtime and feeding. When you finally fall asleep, ten to one your night will be disturbed. Not only do you have to be generous of spirit, you both have to be sacrificial. There are advantages and disadvantages of being a working mother (see above) and the best option for you is whatever makes you happiest. Be prepared, however, for feelings of guilt and inadequacy, but so long as you and your partner are happy, your child will do equally well whether you stay at home or go to work.

3 Choices in childbirth

Only in the last five to eight years have women come to realize that there are choices to be made in childbirth. Until then the majority felt they were entirely in the hands of the medical staff. Partly due to pressure from the women's movement, partly due to enlightenment and flexibility on the part of some medical practitioners, there is a new emphasis on accommodating the needs of individual women, their partners and their babies. Medical routines and interventions are no longer accepted solely on the grounds that they are customary because they make the doctor's job easier, instead the priority has switched to the comfort and happiness of the mother and baby. This is how it should be; it is a pity this change in the way childbirth is approached didn't occur earlier.

TAKING RESPONSIBILITY

A number of women are disappointed by their experience of childbirth; not the birth itself but the way it's conducted, the way they're treated, their inability to get what they want and inadequate help with sorting out their problems. If you are going to have the kind of birth you want, you must first know yourself, know what you want and be explicit in stating your desires. Second, you have to be aware of your options. The way you can achieve this is to read, ask questions, write off to various associations (see p. 229) for information and guidance, be somewhat more self-assertive than you might have been in the past and make sure not to accept anything unless you feel entirely happy about it. Third, you are going to have to learn to communicate. It's all very well having decided in your own head what you would like to happen but if you can't tell others, your hopes will never be realized. It's a good idea to jot things down on paper, to set things out in a logical way. You've got to find the determination and assertiveness to speak out. If you haven't a lot of self-confidence, use a good friend, or better still your partner, for moral support whenever you have to face a frightening situation.

One aim of this chapter is to make it easy for you to plan the kind of childbirth you would like after assessing your own emotional and physical needs. Another aim is to give you the confidence to speak authoritatively in all discussions with your doctor. You are going to have to take a lot of responsibility for yourself and not allow decisions to be made over your head.

To determine your preferences and thoughts you must ask yourself questions such as what would your ideal labor be like, and whether or not you want to be oblivious to the pain and sensations of childbirth.

WHERE TO HAVE YOUR BABY

The two important elements in your choice are whether you want a medically managed or a natural childbirth and whether you want to have your baby at home or in a hospital. Passionate advocates of hospital high-technology births say that this is the only way to ensure that mother and baby will be well looked after if an emergency occurs. At the other extreme natural childbirth advocates are equally forceful in supporting their methods. Some women feel that only in a hospital will they have the security they need. Other women wish to be surrounded by hearth and home when they give birth to their baby.

At home

For women having a normal pregnancy and a normal delivery, home birth can be an attractive option. At one time medical opinion was almost 100 per cent in favor of a hospital delivery being safer but studies have shown that women are much happier at home. If you choose home birth, you will be delivered by a Certified Nurse Midwife, who also attends you throughout pregnancy.

Maternity center or birthing center

This is for women having a normal pregnancy and a normal delivery. A Certified Nurse Midwife attends you throughout pregnancy; you deliver at the maternity center in a homelike environment, with little or no medical intervention (unless it becomes necessary – at which point you are transferred to an affiliate hospital). You may have several birth attendants if you desire, and may deliver in whatever position you choose. Maternity centers also provide a complete program of childbirth and infantcare classes. Fees are much lower than for a hospital birth. Unfortunately few maternity centers exist nationwide.

Alternative birthing room

A number of progressive hospitals have an alternative birth-center, a homelike room in which a woman considered "low-risk" can deliver with little or no medical intervention (see p. 54). Some hospitals employ Certified Nurse Midwives in their birthing rooms; others use obstetric nurses and obstetricians. Where they exist, these rooms are very popular;

Maternity clinic within a hospital

In some clinics you are looked after prenatally by a Certified Nurse Midwife, who may also deliver you. But it is more likely in a hospital clinic that you are attended by several doctors in rotation, so that you don't know in advance who will deliver you.

Clinic outside the hospital

Prenatal care is offered in a community-oriented setting.

Getting information

Spend some time finding out where and how you are going to have the baby. One of the first things you should do is talk to your family doctor. He or she will be able to give you quite a lot of information about what is available in your locality and the various people that you might get in touch with. At the same time talk to nurse-midwives in your area. More and more women are opting for midwife-supervised births since midwife-supervised pregnancy and labor guarantees the one factor that most women desire and which is missing from many hospital pregnancies – continuity of care. The same midwife who sees you during your prenatal visits will probably attend you during the birth. This in itself gives confidence and helps you to relax. Ask friends and neighbors about their birth experiences and recommendations.

HOME BIRTH

There are advantages to having your baby at home if your pregnancy is straightforward and your labor is going to be normal. First of all you keep the responsibility for your child's birth. It is you who leads the way, the other people around you support and help you. You avoid also the travel to the hospital when you are already in labor as well as being moved from room to room once you get there. You will certainly avoid unnecessary medical intervention, and you will have the same midwife throughout pregnancy and at delivery. Starting off breastfeeding is nearly always more successful in the home environment.

You will feel relaxed if you don't have to worry about what your other children are doing.

Mobility

One of the greatest advantages is that you can move around just as you want. Most women find it more comfortable being mobile (see p. 52); it also helps the uterus to work better and keeps the oxygen to the baby at peak level. Sometimes the oxygen supply to the baby is reduced when the mother is lying flat (see p. 53).

Family group

By staying at home you will avoid unhappiness caused by family separation. Probably the greatest advantage is that you and your baby can stay together for those first minutes and hours after the birth. It is important for your partner too, because it is during this time that the first emotional and physical bonding (see p. 202) with the baby begins to develop.

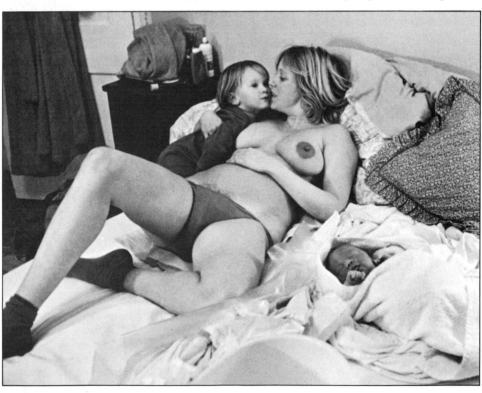

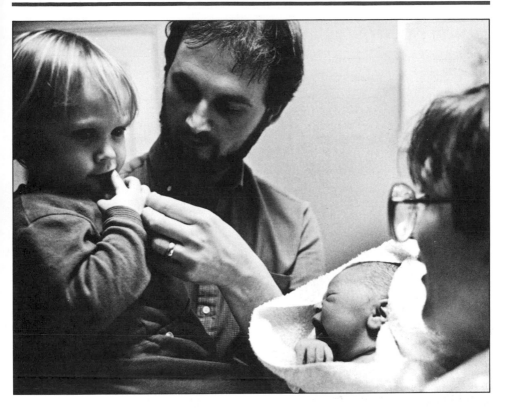

Home birth helps your other children to see birth as a normal part of life and to see the baby as soon as she is born.

Confidence

You'll probably feel confident and relaxed because you're in a familiar place, and this is an advantage to everyone around you. Emotional well-being can definitely affect the function of the uterus. The birth just goes better if you're feeling happy. You'll also avoid the possibility of cross-infection from the medical staff and other mothers and babies who are around you in the hospital. By being at home you will avoid many aspects of the hospital care that you may find distasteful. Their absence will be a bonus.

Organizing a home birth

The first step is to consult your doctor and ask whether or not he or she will provide maternity care for a home birth. You may have to find someone else to look after you during pregnancy. Do this as soon as your pregnancy is diagnosed. If there isn't a doctor in your area who attends home births, call your local hospital to get the names of midwives who practice locally. Or you might write the American College of Nurse-Midwives, 1012 Fourteenth St., N.W., Suite 801, Washington, D.C. 20005.

Because pregnancy is an emotional time, you will want to be attended by someone who can give you emotional support along with technical expertise. Many doctors and midwives will see you briefly for no charge; but call and find out in advance. Don't be afraid, too, of changing doctors during pregnancy. If you are unhappy with your doctor, this can affect your birth experience. Your goal is to be attended by someone you like and trust.

HOSPITAL BIRTH

The decision to have a hospital birth is made for some women because of their physical condition or their obstetric history. Others prefer the medical setting of the hospital. Whether you need or want a hospital birth, before you decide on a particular hospital, there are many questions that you may want to ask and areas that you may want clarified.

☐ Can my partner stay with me all the time and after the baby is delivered? If he can't, can a friend?

☐ If I need a Cesarean section, can my partner or a friend be with me?

☐ May I walk around during labor if everything is okay?

☐ May I choose the position in which I can give birth?

☐ Do I have to be shaved?

☐ Do I have to have an enema or a suppository?

☐ Do women have their waters broken as a routine?

☐ What percentage of women do you induce in this hospital?

☐ How many women have electronic fetal monitoring?

☐ What percentage of women in this hospital have an episiotomy?

☐ What percentage of women have forceps delivery in this hospital?

☐ Can I arrange to have no drugs for pain relief in this hospital?

☐ When a Cesarean birth is planned how many women have epidural anesthesia and how many have general anesthesia?

☐ Can I have as much time as I want to cuddle the baby after delivery if possible?

☐ If I have a Cesarean section can I and/or the father hold the baby afterwards?

☐ May I have my baby with me throughout the 24 hours?

☐ May I breastfeed on demand, including during the night?

☐ Is there free visiting time?

☐ Will my partner be allowed to help with bathing and changing?

☐ Is it possible to arrange a 12-hour or a 24-hour discharge?

How long?

Your hospital stay can be as short as 12 hours. A fairly standard stay is 48 hours or it can be as long as 8–10 days for your first baby. However, it is your right to discharge yourself from the hospital, on your own responsibility, at any time, although you may have pressure put upon you to stay. If you have adequate support and help and there are no complications with you and your baby, there is no reason why you should not go home.

WHY A HOSPITAL DELIVERY

There are good reasons for having a hospital delivery:

● If your medical background includes heart disease, kidney disease, high blood pressure, tuberculosis, asthma, diabetes, serious anemia, obesity or epilepsy.

● If your previous deliveries have included a stillbirth, breech presentation, a transverse or oblique lie (that is if the baby is lying sideways in the pelvis), premature labor before the 37th week of pregnancy, placental insufficiency where the placenta failed to nourish the baby adequately, a difficult forceps delivery or a retained placenta.

● If the following obstetric reasons apply in your case: the baby is too big to pass through the pelvis; true postmaturity; you have toxemia; you are carrying twins; you have bleeding from the vagina late in pregnancy; the placenta is lying in the lower part of the uterus (placenta previa); there is excessive water around the baby; you are an RH negative mother and tests have shown that there are sufficient antibodies in your blood to harm the baby; you have scarring of the uterus because of previous Cesarean sections; or you are over 35 years old and it is your first baby.

Choosing a birth assistant

If you want your partner to be as closely involved with the pregnancy and birth of your child as is possible, he is the natural choice for a birth assistant. He can be the most loving and supportive midwife. His involvement from the beginning will improve your communication in preparation for childbirth. He will be with you during the classes; and you can even do relaxation exercises together.

At the time of labor and delivery your partner is the person who cares for you and gives you most attention. The medical staff are there to support the two of you.

Most women gain reassurance from having their partner with them at their hospital birth.

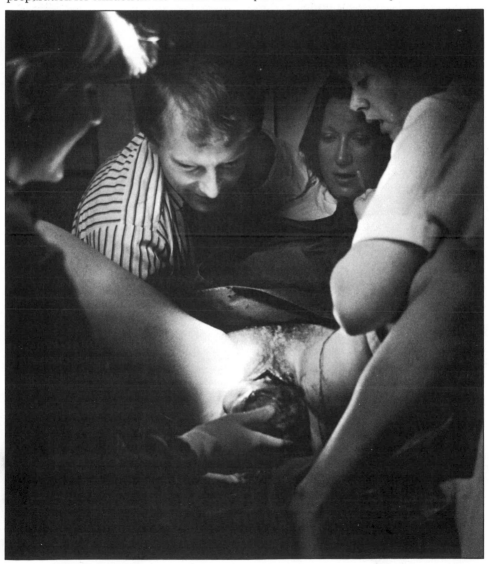

Your partner will give you encouragement and information about what is going on. Childbirth educators spend time preparing couples to cope with the hospital routines and regulations and to improve their relationships with medical staff.

Certified nurse-midwife

This is a registered nurse with additional training who specializes in normal pregnancy. She will follow your pregnancy from prenatal check-ups to delivery to postpartum care. She will stay with you as coach and support throughout your labor, and tends to avoid medical interventions if possible. However, not every hospital will allow a certified nurse-midwife to attend you during labor, so you should check up on the hospital policy.

Obstetrician/gynecologist

Obstetricians vary widely in their approaches to a hospital birth, and you should select yours carefully by asking about matters that concern you (see p. 46).

Family practice physician

Ask the same questions you would ask the obstetrician.

After the birth, you will both feel that you have achieved something miraculous together.

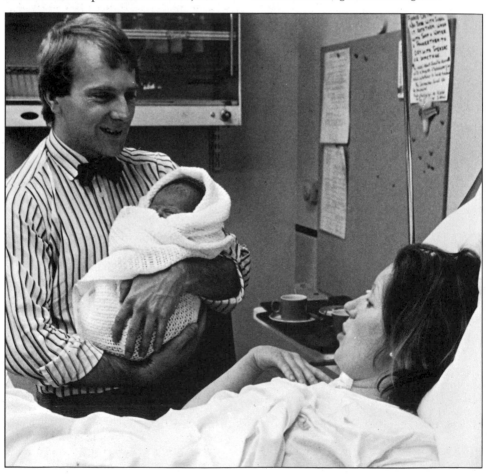

NATURAL CHILDBIRTH

Not surprisingly, most women can and have succeeded with natural childbirth. There are many different reasons for wanting to have your child "naturally" – without fear, unnecessary medical intervention and in a calm atmosphere – just as there are women with varying degrees of commitment to these ends. There are several methods to choose from which offer different approaches and can fit different personalities. Many childbirth classes have taken what they consider to be the best points of several of them to use as their own. Originally, however, there was a pure form of each method.

There is really no one natural way. Whichever way you choose you need to prepare yourself mentally and physically; you could do this informally in your own home with your family and with your partner, as well as in classes. Remember there is no one particular approach that is best for everyone: whatever you do, follow your own feelings.

Grantly Dick-Read

In his book *Childbirth without Fear*, first published in the 1940s, Dr Grantly Dick-Read brought the principles of natural childbirth to public attention. His philosophy was to try to lessen and eliminate fear and tension, and the pain which resulted from these emotions, through proper education and emotional support. The Grantly Dick-Read method will teach you how to cope with tension but lays strong emphasis on the fact that knowledge allays fear and prevents tension, which in turn controls pain. To help you do this there are courses of instruction that include breathing exercises and breathing control and relaxation of muscles (see p. 131), information on what to expect in a normal situation and what you can do to help yourself. This method also teaches you to look for support in the form of guidance, reassurance and sympathy and aims to prepare you for parenthood too.

Psychoprophylaxis

This involves training in breathing methods as a preparation for labor. The techniques were pioneered in Russia and introduced in the West by Dr Fernand Lamaze. The Lamaze method is by far the most popular in the United States. It encourages the woman to take responsibility for herself, and to work as a team with her partner, friends and teachers. The woman must prepare her body in the last few months of pregnancy with special exercises and she has to train her mind to respond automatically to each type of contraction she will feel in labor. She sees herself as a rational member of the childbirth team, consisting usually of four people – herself, her partner, the doctor and the nurse. The partner acts as "coach" and as emotional support. He is expected to attend the course with her and co-operate with her at home on the conditioning exercises and to coach, coax and comfort her throughout labor and delivery.

The Leboyer philosophy

This relies on several basic precepts and relates more to the baby than the mother and her progress throughout labor. Dr Frederick Leboyer, in his book *Birth without Violence*, states that the newborn baby is extremely sensitive through its skin, its ears, its eyes – in fact that it reflects all the emotions surrounding it – anger, anxiety, impatience, calm etc. For that reason he believes that all stimulation to the baby at the moment of birth should be minimized with low lights, few sounds, little handling, and with immersion in water at body heat so that the baby's entry into the world is as little different from its life in the womb as possible.

This teaching is in fact not entirely in line with the physiology of what occurs at the moment of birth for the baby. It is contact with air at a temperature different from body temperature that makes the baby take its first gulp of air starting the initial crucial function of the lungs as well as causing the baby's blood circulation to change from a fetal one to a mature one. Without these two things occurring a baby's life is in jeopardy.

It is also simply not true to say that a baby's hearing is so sensitive that it is disturbed by noises around it. The sound of the uterine vessels within the womb are akin to a loud vacuum cleaner. Leboyer also believes that the mother is an "enemy and a monster" to the child, driving it and crushing it within the birth passage. He likens her to a torturer. Many women object to this view as it minimizes, even diminishes, the role of the mother.

Dr Leboyer believes that the baby should not be touched by foreign materials but by human skin. The ideal place for the baby is to be laid face down on the mother's abdomen and covered by her arms. It has been proven by experiment that this is far more efficient in preventing the baby from losing heat than overhead heaters. Research has shown that the baby is able to clear mucus from its respiratory passages more efficiently when lying face down on its mother's stomach than with a suction tube.

Leboyer suggests that the curtains and blinds in the delivery room are drawn and the lights are dimmed. Some medical authorities object to this as they say it is not possible to assess the baby's condition in a dim light.

Very few hospitals practice the pure Leboyer method, but many practice Leboyer-based birth. It seemed to me on first reading Leboyer that all he had done was to formalize what midwives had been doing, in principle, for years. It is still fairly difficult to find pure Leboyer methods, even adapted ones, being used in modern teaching hospitals where the accent is on speed and high technology. Medical authorities have been slow to adopt Leboyer because research has shown that Leboyer babies appear to receive no extra benefit compared to others, though "Leboyer mothers" may feel they do.

Dr Michel Odent

At his clinic in France Michel Odent places the mother in an environment which is cosy and home-like, giving her complete freedom to act as she wishes and encouraging her to reach a new level of animal consciousness where she forgets her inhibitions and returns to a rather primitive biological state. Dr Odent believes that the high levels of endorphins, nature's natural narcotics, should be allowed to have full rein in the mother's body. He logically argues that if a woman is given pain killers and analgesics her endorphins are cut off, thus depriving her of natural pain relief.

I have visited Dr Odent's clinic, discussed his philosophies with him, seen women give birth in different ways, all subjectively suited to them, and talked to them about their experiences. Dr Odent's delivery room is itself like a womb. The furnishings are all soft, there are no chairs, just piles of cushions on which women can lie and recline. The lights are fairly dim, there is music, and the whole atmosphere is relaxing. A woman who goes into labor is allowed to sit, walk, stand, eat and drink and do whatever she wants. Women are not interfered with in any way and can take up whatever position is most comfortable for them at any stage of the labor. Left to their own devices many women take up a position on all fours which seems to help the pain. Later on in birth many stand up or semi-squat so that the force of gravity can help them, a natural thing to do which most primitive tribes practice. Odent encourages the supported squatting position where he, or the woman's partner, stands behind her, takes her weight underneath her armpits and upper arm and allows her to bend her knees and place her weight on her partner's arm. There is a bath in the next room which sometimes helps women to relax and they are encouraged to try it. If they very much want to stay there, Dr Odent is quite happy to deliver the baby into the water of the bath if that's what happens.

Dr Odent has low rates of episiotomy, forceps and Cesarean section. The supported squat position is the one which prevents severe perineal tears during delivery. Because the mother has been in an upright position when the baby emerges she remains sitting upright with the cord still intact and the baby in her lap. The baby immediately smells the mother's skin and it is thought that this is important to the baby in establishing breastfeeding. Within a few seconds most mothers instinctively lift the baby up and place it at the breast. No partner needs to be told to encircle the mother and the baby with his own body and arms. Most are very moved and many cry. But the three people are enjoying very close human communion.

The yogic method

This is for those who already practice yoga. During birth a woman should concentrate her awareness on being totally at one with what is happening to her. Through yogic methods she is able to control her awareness according to her capacity and tolerance, so at some times she is able to distract herself from the contractions and at others be totally involved in them. She may use meditation and chanting and the support of yoga groups' spiritual participation. Practitioners in the yogic methods believe that a woman can handle childbirth in a mature and serene way. Yogic childbirth education helps in the belief that a woman has the ability to create or destroy her own pain, similarly her own joy, during birth.

NURSING AND MEDICAL PROCEDURES

Not every hospital practices the procedures that follow but many of them are common. No-one in these hospitals seems to question their justification or their necessity or even whether childbirth would be better, safer or more comfortable without them. I feel that they ought to be challenged so I am giving you information so that you can come to some decision yourself as to whether you think certain medical procedures are justified and if you'd like them for yourself.

Enemas

These are given to clear out the bowel, usually in the form of warm soapy water inserted into your rectum, the rationale being that the bowel once emptied will leave as much room as possible for the baby and spare the woman the embarrassment of pushing out faeces as the baby's head is delivered. Besides being of questionable logic, they are hardly needed if nature is allowed to take its course. The onset of labor is very often accompanied by several bowel movements as the intestinal muscles start to contract in sympathy with uterine muscle. Routine enemas discount the fact that you may

have just emptied your bowels and also that you may not have eaten recently and so your bowel is empty. Suppositories, slower-acting capsules that irritate the lining of the rectum, are sometimes used. Some medical practitioners believe that an enema makes the uterine contractions longer and brings on the labor more quickly. One of the side effects of this is that if you get a profound reaction to the enema, you will be rushing to the toilet to empty your bowels and this may upset you and make you anxious. Find out if enemas are routine in the delivery ward that you are entering. There are simply no grounds for giving a routine enema if you've just emptied your bowels. So you might like to ask that an enema would not be given under these circumstances.

Shaving of the pubic hair

This is quite unnecessary (unless you are having a Cesarean section), but even so it is shaved off routinely in many hospitals, on the grounds that hair is dirty and harbors bacteria, making it impossible to sterilize the perineum. Shaving of pubic hair will therefore reduce the possibility of infection. However, the actual reason for shaving is that it makes the repair of the episiotomy or a tear easier for the doctor. So if you are in a hospital unit where episiotomies are the rule, shaving of the pubic hair is almost certainly routine.

The real question to be asked is whether shaving does reduce the incidence of infection. The results of careful studies suggest that the reverse is true: shaving increases infection. In the light of this it seems perfectly reasonable for you to object to having the pubic area shaved. In support of this you can quote excellent studies which have shown that a simplified method of preparing the pubic area is more effective in cutting down infection than shaving. The vulva is wiped with gauze to remove any mucus or blood and the area is sprayed with an antiseptic, so eliminating any chance of infection.

Confinement to bed

There is absolutely no good reason why a woman should be confined to bed during labor except that it has become a customary part of obstetric practice, it fits in more easily with ward routine and there is resistance to change. It is quite unnatural, not to say uncomfortable, for a woman to remain in one position during labor. But the majority of women who go into a hospital are expected to stay in bed principally because of the electronic fetal monitors (see p. 190). This implies that only a few limited positions are available to her. The same applies to the delivery table, which imposes on a woman an automatic and inefficient position for delivery. An excellent study done in Latin America has shown that in a group of mothers having their first baby the length of labor in those who were allowed to move around as they wanted to was only two thirds as long as that of the women who were confined to bed. When all mothers were considered, the mobile group were 25 per cent quicker in producing their babies than those who did not move around.

The study also found that 95 per cent of mothers who are left to themselves prefer to be upright and are more comfortable when upright. When mothers spend time in different positions in labor they report less pain and greater comfort when sitting, standing, kneeling or squatting.

The study concludes that in normal spontaneous labor women who are allowed to assume a vertical position have an easier progress through labor, shorten its duration and have less discomfort and pain. In light of all this, it seems unreasonable to deny women who are having normal labors the right to choose the position or positions that they find most comfortable during the first and second stage of labor, since this is also likely to be the most advantageous position for them in terms of their pelvic shape and the position of the baby. I don't accept the argument which says that it is more convenient for the midwife or doctor if the woman lies flat. It is the doctor who should fit in with the patient.

Positions for delivery

Before the end of the seventeenth century when labor rooms were the province of women, no one considered that a woman's normal behavior should be interfered with. She was allowed to move about as she wanted, take up any position that she felt was comfortable, eat and drink as she wished and assume her chosen position for delivering the baby. Then doctors invaded the delivery room and at that time all

Delivery position
It is more efficient to give birth in a semi-vertical position. The force of gravity helps to push the baby down and out rather than into the bed if you are lying flat on your back.

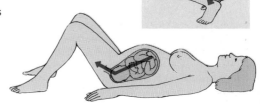

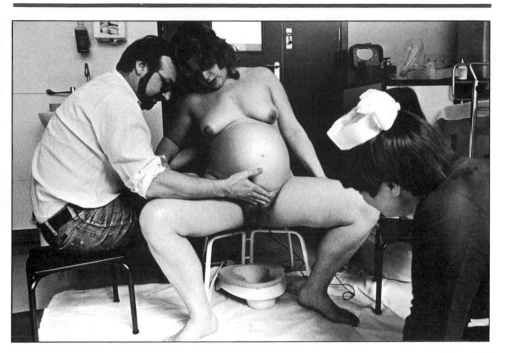

Birthing stools allow you to be in a vertical position where the force of gravity can help to push the baby out.

doctors were men. A French doctor at the royal court proposed that women should lie on their backs in preference to using upright positions and birthing stools to make vaginal examinations and obstetric maneuvers easier, not because it might benefit the mother or the baby.

It is natural for a woman to take up a semi-vertical position for delivery of the baby, not just because it's comfortable but because it is mechanically most efficient. When she is upright the uterine contractions are aiming downwards, pushing the baby out towards the floor. When a woman pushes she strains downwards in the same direction and most importantly the force of gravity helps too. When a woman lies on her back, the uterine contractions push the baby into the bed and not down the birth canal so the added advantage of the force of gravity is lost. The result is that the recumbent

woman has to push her baby up and against the force of gravity. This not only prolongs labor but makes the possibility of all complications, including the need for an episiotomy, greater.

A position adopted in many hospital units is one involving the use of knee braces. This is called the lithotomy

DISADVANTAGES OF LYING ON YOUR BACK FOR DELIVERY
If you lie on your back:
- your blood pressure may drop, thus reducing the amount of blood and oxygen to the baby
- pain is greater in this position than in a vertical one
- there is a greater need for an episiotomy
- there is an increased chance of a forceps delivery
- it inhibits spontaneous delivery of the placenta
- there is a greater possibility of low back strain in this position.

position. This has no science or logic. Some progressive obstetrics centers have come round to realize this and have abandoned this outdated position. Question the practices in your center and see if it would be possible for you to opt to have your baby in one of the positions outlined on p. 171. If you cannot and you are told that you must have your baby in the recumbent position, you may wish to reconsider your decision to have your baby in that center.

Withholding food and drink

In many cultures a woman in labor is encouraged to take food and drink from time to time, particularly herbal teas, to keep her strength up; withholding food and drink is a relatively new practice. The stomach seems to close down, however, and any food taken during labor may be vomited up. There is absolutely no rationale for allowing a woman nothing during labor; in fact often a woman has a sudden demand for energy and for this she needs sugar. If sugar isn't available she starts to use fat stores as a form of energy.

The reason given for withholding food and drink from women in labor is that they may need an emergency general anesthetic. But this is not a good enough reason to withhold food from all women rather than only those who are at risk of needing a surgical procedure. Many women in labor don't want to eat but most of them require fluids, particularly as labor advances and fluids are lost through sweating, so water or ice chips should be given, in my opinion, when requested. Otherwise an intravenous drip will be set up to administer glucose solution directly to the mother, bypassing the stomach and increasing the medical intervention in her labor.

Moving to a delivery room

Ideally labor should proceed smoothly in peaceful, undisturbed surroundings. Any disruption may adversely affect its course. It is in the transition stage that you often find yourself in the most stressful part of labor. Yet at this point in hospitals you must go through the physical and emotional upheaval of getting off one bed, onto a stretcher, and being wheeled from one room to another.

In most hospital centers there is a special room which is designed for delivery and which has the style and atmosphere of an operating room, since it must sometimes function as such. You will have your baby on a narrow table that is usually suspended on a central column which is raised and lowered pneumatically. During your prenatal clinic ask about the delivery room and explore if there are any alternatives to this environment. If there aren't, take a look around. You may be able to bring in something to help you. If they have a tape machine, ask if you can bring some tapes.

There is no real justification for the rigidity on the part of nursing and medical attendants; their sad lack of imagination shows little feeling for what the mother is experiencing. I can see no reason why it is necessary for a woman in normal labor to have to give birth in a delivery room rather than a homey labor room which is equipped with good lighting, oxygen in some form and suction apparatus to clear out the baby's air passages if necessary.

ALTERNATIVE BIRTHING ROOM
Some progressive hospitals have set up alternative birthing rooms which have a home-like environment within the hospital where a woman can deliver almost exactly as if she were at home but with medical facilities on tap should either she or her baby need them. There is no uncomfortable break in the progression of labor to a separate delivery room and you don't have to lie on a delivery table surrounded by clinical paraphernalia. For many women the alternative birthing room is an ideal compromise between a technological, de-personalized hospital birth and a birth at home.

CHOOSING HOW TO FEED

The most important aspect of infant feeding is feeding the infant. Most babies thrive whether they are breast or bottle fed. Given that as a basis, there are other considerations. Your preference cannot be overlooked. Feeding will be most successful if you are happy with the method you have chosen, and in order to make a choice and exercise an option you have to be aware of the pros and cons of breast and bottle or a combination of both. And you must think about what is best for the baby. There's little doubt that where the baby's well-being is concerned, breastfeeding is superior.

Advantages of breastfeeding

☐ A good reason for breastfeeding is that it's the natural thing to do. Most women have a natural urge to breastfeed, and there are very few women who are not physically equipped to breastfeed. No matter how small the breasts, they are going to be able to produce enough milk to feed and sustain the baby. Even women whose nipples are inverted can, with early diagnosis, breastfeed their babies (see p. 83). It's natural for a mother to feel proud that her baby is being fed on food that she provides; to crave the physical nearness and pleasure that breastfeeding offers; and to enjoy knowing that you are helping a close relationship to develop between you and your child.

☐ Breastfed babies are less liable to illness than bottle-fed ones (this was shown in a much quoted survey done in 1948). There are fewer cases of gastro-enteritis, chest infection and measles. All the mother's antibodies to bacterial and viral infections are present in the colostrum, the first milk made by the breasts and present in the breasts from the fifth month of pregnancy. In the first few days of life therefore, when the baby is taking only the high-protein colostrum, she is living under the umbrella of her mother's antibodies. They have a protective effect in the intestine but also,

as they're absorbed straight into the baby's system unchanged, they form an important part of the baby's own protection against infections. Take the example of a mother who has antibodies to poliomyelitis in her own body; because those antibodies appear in her colostrum, it's not possible to infect her baby with the poliomyelitis virus while she's being wholly breastfed. The antibodies in the baby's gut will kill the virus before it can do any harm. Besides that, human milk is antibacterial because it contains substances that destroy bacteria. Even though these substances are present in cow's milk, a bottle-fed baby is not protected in the same way because the antibodies are inactivated when the cow's milk is heated.

☐ Human breast milk is the best source of food for a human baby; it has just the right amount of minerals and proteins. Cow's milk, which is for calves, has a higher percentage of protein and a high content of casein, which is the least digestible part of it and is passed out in the stool in the form of curds. Human milk contains just the right amount of sodium for a newborn baby. This is important because the immature kidneys of the infant are unable to deal with high levels of sodium in the blood. Cow's milk contains more sodium than human milk. While human milk and cow's milk contain the same amount of fat, the droplets in human milk are smaller and more digestible. Breast milk fat is high in polyunsaturates and low in cholesterol, and it may therefore protect against heart disease in later life. Breast milk contains more sugar (lactose) than cow's milk and the mineral and vitamin content is different.

☐ Breastfeeding is good for the figure. Research has shown that a woman loses most of the fat she's accumulated during pregnancy if she breastfeeds. If you don't feed your baby yourself, you may have more difficulty returning to your pre-pregnancy weight.

55

☐ It's a common fallacy that the breasts lose their shape and firmness through breastfeeding. This is not so. The changes that occur in the breasts are a consequence of becoming pregnant, not of producing milk or feeding your baby. Breastfeeding also causes the release of the hormone oxytocin which encourages the uterus to shrink to its non-pregnant size, hastening the return to normal of the pelvis and your waistline.

☐ The sheer convenience of breastfeeding also mustn't be ignored.

The important elements of choosing how to feed your baby are that you and the baby are both happy and that the baby is thriving.

☐ Bonding should occur between mother and baby automatically if you breastfeed. When a baby is at the breast, her face is close to her mother's face, and even a newborn baby can focus at this distance. The act of making eye contact, and smiling at your baby as she sucks, helps to create a physical and emotional bond between mother and baby which is hardly broken for the rest of their lives.

Disadvantages of breastfeeding

One of the often quoted disadvantages of breastfeeding is that it curtails social activity. This need not necessarily be so if you can manage to express off sufficient milk manually or with a breast pump (see

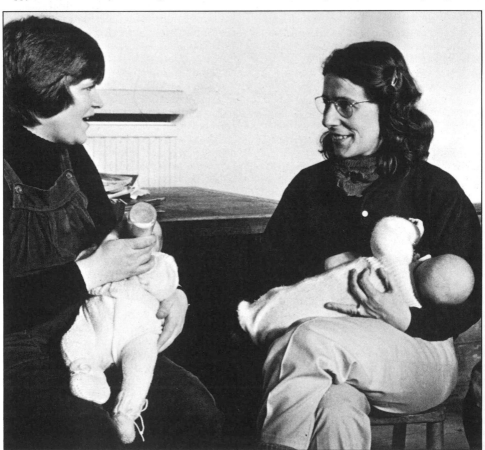

p. 224) to serve the baby's needs while you're absent. You can bottle your own breast milk in sterile bottles and store them in the refrigerator or freezer, and your babysitter can give the bottle to your baby on your behalf. Remember, even if you only feed your baby for two weeks, that's better than not breastfeeding at all and gives your baby a flying start in life. Incidentally, one of the advantages of expressing some of your milk into bottles is that your partner can become involved with the feeding routine too.

Bottle feeding

☐ As there are no real arguments against breastfeeding, a converse of this is that there are no arguments in favour of bottle feeding. However, for you in your particular circumstances with your particular predilections, breastfeeding may not be a feasible or workable alternative, in which case bottle feeding will be your choice. If it is, don't feel that your child is getting second best.

☐ Babies thrive and are perfectly happy being bottle fed, and always remember that your baby needs your love and care more than she needs your breast milk. Bottle feeding, love and attention are an excellent option for any baby.

☐ There will be certain mothers who don't have any option but to bottle feed. These are women who may be taking drugs in the long term for a medical condition, such as epilepsy, which needs barbiturates to keep it under control, and chronic depression, for which antidepressants are prescribed. You may become seriously ill and need admission to a hospital. If physically you're not in a fit state to breastfeed, then you should not. If you have to take any medicines regularly, discuss whether or not they appear in the milk and what the possible effects will be on breastfeeding and your baby. Quite often it's possible to change drugs for nursing mothers.

☐ Some handicapped babies or babies with physical abnormalities such as cleft palate or deformity of the jaw and mouth may not be able to suck successfully and will have to be bottle fed.

☐ If breastfeeding gets off to a difficult start and your milk supply never becomes established, the baby will fail to thrive and you should opt to bottle feed.

☐ Some women have a strong physical revulsion against breastfeeding and find it a tiresome chore. A woman who feels revulsion very strongly will be under stress, and this may interfere both with milk production and milk flow. If you feel that your baby is not getting enough, these negative messages will reinforce your dislike of breastfeeding. Do try to talk over your feelings before the birth of your baby with a sympathetic friend or your doctor and do involve your baby's father.

☐ One of the main advantages of bottle feeding is that your partner can be involved in feeding your baby from the outset. It also means that you can work out a shared feeding schedule which gives you enough time for rest, unbroken sleep and time off for yourself.

☐ One of the questionable advantages of bottle feeding is that babies sleep longer between feedings during the first weeks. This could be because the casein content of cow's milk is higher than that of human milk and takes longer to digest.

☐ With bottle feeding, you can see exactly how much milk your baby has taken, which when the baby is very young can be most reassuring.

Disadvantages of bottle feeding

The spit-up from a bottlefed baby has rather an unpleasant smell, as do the stools. The other major problem is allergy, which occurs if the baby proves to be sensitive to the alien protein in the cow's milk. There are soya substitutes for babies with allergies and those babies in families with a history of asthma or eczema are advised to try to breastfeed or use these substitutes.

The sterilization of bottlefeeding equipment and the careful preparation of formula is time consuming compared to the accessibility of breast milk.

4 Prenatal care

Prenatal care is the key to healthy mothers, happy pregnancies and thriving babies. It's now accepted by most doctors that the one way in which we can improve the statistics on childbirth is through early and vigorous prenatal care.

For most women their prenatal care is smooth and happy. By talking to other mothers and to doctors and midwives, you can find out more and more about pregnancy and birth, which should help to reassure you and make you feel more confident about forthcoming events. Much prenatal care is routine, but asking questions and exploring the different circumstances in which you can have your baby will help you to plan ahead to get the kind of labor and birth you want.

GOING TO THE DOCTOR

As soon as you suspect or know that you are pregnant, go to see your doctor. He or she will ask you for the date of the first day of your last menstrual period (LMP). It is from this day that the pregnancy is measured. Depending on how far your pregnancy is advanced, your doctor will perform some kind of pregnancy test – either a urine test (see p. 36) or an internal examination if you are at least eight weeks pregnant. He or she will confirm the pregnancy even if you have already used a home kit yourself.

There is a blood test that is so sensitive, pregnancy can be detected before you miss your first period. Your doctor can also date your pregnancy with this test. A blood sample will be drawn by the doctor for laboratory analysis. This is not available in all centers but it has the advantage of alerting you to your pregnancy so that you can watch your nutritional intake and stop taking any drugs at this vital time.

The first visit

Once your pregnancy has been confirmed, your doctor will take a medical and family history as well as do a physical examination. In addition, you will want to state in general terms what your preferences for birth are going to be (see pp. 42–57), so give the subject some thought before your appointment. These preferences may conflict with your doctor's desire to stick to routines and procedures that he or she is used to and is not willing to change. If you feel strongly about some aspect of your pregnancy or labor, but fear that you may be browbeaten into accepting something else, take along your partner or an articulate friend for moral support. Their presence alone may give you the strength to state your case and stick to it.

Use your doctor as a source of information: ask for a list of recommended books to read, pamphlets to send off for and the names of nurse-midwives to talk to. If it's your first baby and you'd like to talk to another mother, ask for the names of other patients.

Your time at the doctor's office can be spent talking about pregnancy with the other mothers.

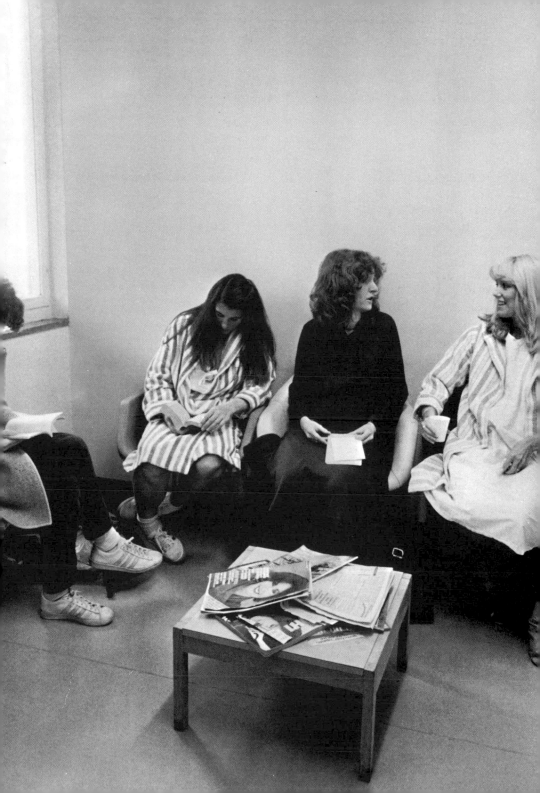

ROUTINE PRENATAL TESTS

Name	Purpose	Significance
Height and shoe size	To assess size of pelvis and pelvic outlet.	Very small shoe size or height can suggest a small pelvic outlet and consequently maybe a difficult delivery.
Weight	To follow growth of fetus. Try to wear the same weight of clothing so your weight doesn't fluctuate unnecessarily.	A loss of weight will be investigated, although this is usual during the first trimester if you suffer from nausea and vomiting. Sudden weight gain may indicate pre-eclampsia (see p. 150).
Breasts	Check for lumps and condition of nipples.	If nipples are retracted and you wish to breastfeed, you will be advised to wear a breast shield (see p. 83), do gentle exercises on the nipples or just wait and see. They may correct themselves during the pregnancy.
Heart, lungs, hair, eyes, teeth, nails	To check on your general physical health.	You may need some special attention and dietary supplements (see p. 101) or just general advice on diet. Dental visits will be encouraged.
Legs and hands	To look for varicose veins and any swelling (edema) in the ankles, hands or fingers.	Cases of extreme puffiness can be a sign of pre-eclampsia (see p. 150). Advice on what to do about varicose veins will be given (see p. 142).
Urine (MSU)	To test for kidney infection. After cleaning the vulva with sterile pads, you pass a sample of urine into a sterile container. Allow the first drops to go into the toilet bowl and collect the mid-stream urine (MSU) only.	An existing kidney infection you may not know you have can develop into a serious condition in pregnancy. You will be treated with antibiotics.
Urine	1. Tests for protein in case your kidneys aren't coping well. 2. Tests for the presence of sugar; if found repeatedly, you may have diabetes. 3. Tests for ketones; if found, it is almost always a sign of diabetes.	1. Protein in urine late in pregnancy is a sign of pre-eclampsia (see p. 150). Bed rest will probably be prescribed. 2. Pregnancy can unmask diabetes (see p. 145), which must be treated and stabilized. It may go away after delivery only to return in later pregnancies. 3. Presence of ketones indicates that the body is short of sugar. You will be given treatment for diabetes. Ketones are, however, rarely found in these tests.
Internal examination	To confirm the pregnancy and to check that the uterus is the size it should be according to the dates. To take a Pap smear to exclude cancer of the cervix. To check for pelvic abnormalities. To check that the cervix is tightly closed.	Excludes problems with the cervix and the pelvic cavity. If cancer test is positive, you will need to discuss the options with the obstetrician. Mention if either you or your partner has ever suffered from genital herpes. This can cause meningitis in the baby. If you have an active infection at the end of pregnancy, you will be delivered by Cesarean section.

Name	Purpose	Significance
Fetal heart beat	To confirm that the fetus is alive and that the heart and heart rate are normal.	If the doctor listens to your baby's heart with a Doppler probe (this listens to the fetal heart with ultrasound vibrations), the sound of the beat will be amplified so you can hear it too.
Abdominal palpation	To assess the height of the fundus (the top of the uterus – see p. 85), and the size and position of the fetus.	Gives a guide to the length of the pregnancy and the lie of the fetus in the womb. This is important if at 32 weeks the fetus has not turned from the breech position to the head first or cephalic position (see p. 161). The doctor may try to turn the baby by a process known as external cephalic version (ECV) (see p. 192).
Blood pressure	This is the measurement of the pressure at which the heart is pumping blood through your body. The test is done to assess if it is normal or not. The reading is made up of two numbers: the top one is the systolic pressure, when the heart contracts, pushes out blood and "beats." This can be heard when the arm band is tightened; the bottom one is the diastolic pressure, the resting pressure between heart beats. A normal BP is 120/70.	Hypertension (high blood pressure) can indicate a number of problems, including pre-eclampsia (see p. 150). Constant checks mean it can be kept under control if it suddenly rises, e.g. above 140/90. May mean bed rest in the hospital if it rises. Any rise in the lower or diastolic figure is cause for concern.
Blood tests	1. To determine your major blood group ABO. 2. To find your RH blood group. 3. To find your hemoglobin level (repeated test). This is a measure of the oxygen-carrying substances in your red blood cells. Normal levels, measured in gm., are between 12 and 14gm. 4. Alpha fetoprotein levels – a special test at 16 weeks. 5. To detect the presence of German measles antibodies. 6. VDRL, Kahn or Wasserman tests for the presence of syphilis. 7. To detect sickle cell disease and thalassemia, both forms of anemia found in dark-skinned people and inhabitants of Mediterranean countries.	1. Blood group needed in case of an emergency transfusion. 2. In case of RH blood incompatability (see p. 150). 3. During pregnancy your hemoglobin level may drop, because pregnant women have more circulating blood (see p. 86), but if it goes below 10gm, treatment for anemia (see p. 144) will be given. Iron and folic acid supplements will raise the hemoglobin level so that more oxygen can be carried to the baby. 4. See p. 67. 5. To find out whether or not you have immunity to rubella, if not you will be warned not to come into contact with German measles during your pregnancy (see p. 24). 6. If you unknowingly have this sexually transmitted infection, it is essential to treat it before week 20 of your pregnancy; after this time it can be passed to the baby. 7. Can affect the baby and the pregnancy. Your blood will be tested for this blood disease if you are from a race which is affected by it. Extra folic acid will be prescribed and in extreme cases of sickle cell, a blood transfusion may be necessary.

The first visit

The purpose of your first visit to the doctor is to give information so that the doctor can judge whether or not your pregnancy and delivery will be normal.

The physical examination

This would probably be the most complete physical examination of your pregnancy. Until the last month, you will most likely not be examined internally again.

- Your height and weight will be measured
- Your blood pressure will be taken
- Your ears, nose and throat will be checked; your heart and lungs listened to;

MEDICAL AND FAMILY HISTORY

At the initial interview you will be asked some or all of the following questions about your relevant medical and past obstetric history:

- your name, age, race, date and place of birth, date of marriage if any
- about your childhood illnesses, and whether or not you have ever been in a hospital or had any serious disease or any surgical operations
- if any illnesses run in your family or your partner's
- whether there are any twins in either family
- whether you used contraceptives, if so what sort and when you stopped
- about your menstrual history, when the periods first started, how long your average cycle is, how many days you bleed and the date of the first day of your last menstrual period
- whether you have any symptoms of pregnancy and what your general state of health is like
- about the births of any other children you may have, or any miscarriages
- whether you are taking any prescriptive medicines or suffer from any allergies
- what work you and your partner do and whether you are still working.

and your breasts and abdomen palpated

- You will have a pelvic examination a) to determine the size and shape of your pelvis; b) to determine the size and shape of your uterus and the age of the fetus; c) to check the health of your reproductive organs; d) to have a Pap smear done to check for cervical cancer
- Your blood will be tested a) to determine your blood group, RH factor, and for antibody screening; b) for a complete blood count; c) to test for rubella; d) to test for syphilis; e) to test for toxoplasmosis
- A urine specimen will be taken a) to test for protein and sugar; b) to test for infection.

Asking questions

An important part of your first visit is getting information. You will want to find out what hospital your doctor admits to, when you should pre-register, and what his fees are. It will also help you to gain confidence in your pregnancy if you express your concerns. While it isn't essential at the first visit, it's a good idea to tell your doctor your preferences for pain relief during labor, whether you want an early discharge from the hospital, and what course of action you would want if the baby was overdue.

Subsequent visits

Your visits will occur every four weeks until the 28th week, every two weeks to the 36th week, and thereafter weekly until you go into labor. You will probably have more blood tests after the 32nd week to confirm that everything is going well. In addition to your weight, blood pressure and urine being checked, the doctor will check the height of the top of the uterus and the rate of the baby's heartbeat, as well as the baby's position.

During the last month you will again have internal examinations. Your doctor will check the baby's position abdominally, and will also check how far the baby's head has descended and the condition of the cervix.

YOUR MONTHLY VISIT

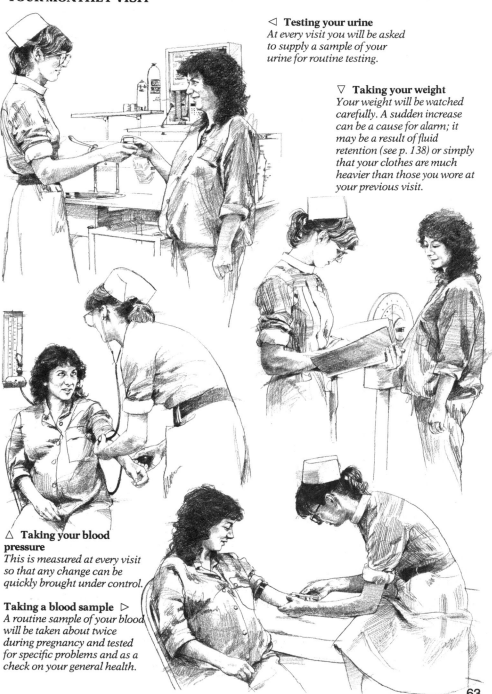

◁ **Testing your urine**
*At every visit you will be asked
to supply a sample of your
urine for routine testing.*

▽ **Taking your weight**
*Your weight will be watched
carefully. A sudden increase
can be a cause for alarm; it
may be a result of fluid
retention (see p. 138) or simply
that your clothes are much
heavier than those you wore at
your previous visit.*

△ **Taking your blood
pressure**
*This is measured at every visit
so that any change can be
quickly brought under control.*

Taking a blood sample ▷
*A routine sample of your blood
will be taken about twice
during pregnancy and tested
for specific problems and as a
check on your general health.*

The older woman

Just as important as the age of the mother is her past medical history, diet and lifestyle (see p. 22). However, at the first prenatal visit, the older first-time mother will be asked many questions, as she is statistically more likely to fall into a group requiring special attention. Once all the questions are answered, problem areas identified and necessary tests performed (see p. 68), prenatal care for the older woman will not differ from the norm.

Childbirth and infantcare classes

For first-time parents in particular, these classes are designed to give confidence and information. They should give you both an understanding of pregnancy and birth and teach you techniques of relaxation, breathing and exercise to prepare you for labor. Separate infantcare classes help you to learn to cope with a small baby. Shop around for the classes in your area that emphasize the aspects of pregnancy and childcare you feel most unsure about. Ask your doctor or midwife for suggestions. Start early so you can get into your chosen class. It is worth attending hospital orientation classes too as they help you to understand the procedures in that hospital and you will be able to look around the delivery room and postnatal wards.

The delivery room will not seem so strange if you familiarize yourself with it at childbirth classes.

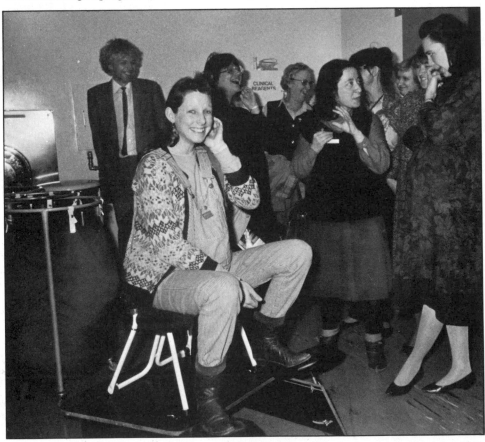

UNDERSTANDING YOUR MEDICAL RECORD

At your prenatal visits, your doctor will record the details of the routine tests and the progress of your pregnancy. He or she may use abbreviations and some of these are explained below. If your doctor uses a term relating to your condition that you don't understand, ask for an explanation.

NAD or nil or a tick	Nothing abnormal discovered in urine.
Alb	Albumin in urine (a name for one of the proteins found in urine).
BP	Blood pressure.
FHH/NH	Fetal heart heard or not heard.
FH	Fetal heart.
FMF	Fetal movements felt.
Ceph.	Cephalic, baby is head down.
Vx	Vertex, the baby is head down.
Br.	Breech, the baby is bottom down.
LMP	Last menstrual period.
EDC	Estimated date of confinement.
Hb	Hemoglobin levels to check for anemia.
Eng/E	Engaged, the baby's head has dropped into the pelvis ready for birth.
NE	Not engaged.
Para O	Woman has had no other children.
Para 1 (etc)	Woman has had one child.
Fe	Iron has been prescribed.
TCA	To come again.

Height of fundus	The height of the top of the uterus. The baby pushes this up as it grows and often the height is used to estimate the length of the pregnancy. Some doctors measure the height of the fundus (from the top of the pubic bone to the top of the uterus) with a tape measure in centimeters. This figure is usually roughly the same as the length of the pregnancy in weeks.
Relation of PP to brim	This is the brim of your pelvis. The presenting part (PP) of the baby to the brim in the later stages of your pregnancy will be the part in the cervix ready to be born first.
PET	Pre-eclamptic toxemia.
Ed.	Edema.
Long L	Longitudinal lie, the baby is parallel to your spine in the womb.
RSA	Right sacrum anterior – the most common breech presentation.
AFP	Alpha fetoprotein.
CS	Cesarean section.
H/T	Hypertension.
MSU	Mid-stream urine sample.
Primipara	First pregnancy.
Multipara	More than one pregnancy.
VE	Vaginal examination.

The lie of the baby
Certain abbreviations describe the way the baby is lying in the womb (see p. 161 and 192): These abbreviations refer to the position of the crown of the baby's head (occiput) in relation to your body; that is whether on the right or left, to the front (anterior) or back (posterior).

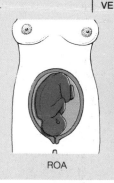
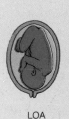
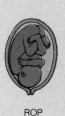
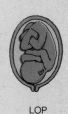

ROA   LOA   ROP   LOP

SPECIAL TESTS

Ultrasound

Ultrasound is very useful as a way of determining the age of the fetus, the position of the placenta and your expected date of delivery. The test works by giving a photographic picture formed by the echoes of sound waves bouncing off different parts of the body of different consistencies. Unlike X-rays, ultrasound can give soft tissue in detail and will print out a very accurate picture to the trained eye of the fetus *in utero* (see below). The picture will be explained to you if you can't understand it.

If your doctor opts for ultrasound, the first scan will be done at about 12–14 weeks and then at any time during pregnancy after that.

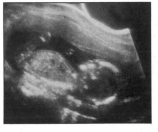

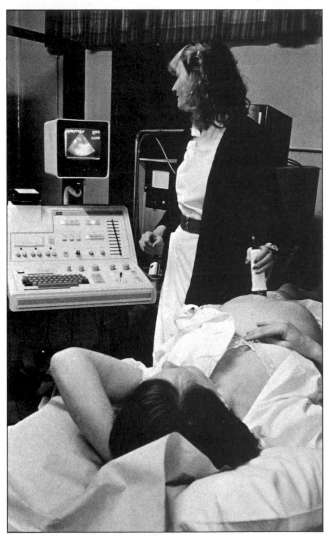

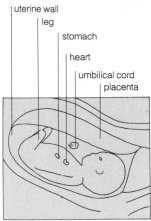

uterine wall
leg
stomach
heart
umbilical cord
placenta

The fetus in utero

It is very exciting to see a picture of your baby in your womb. The shapes may not make much sense to you so ask the technician to point out the head, limbs and the baby's organs. The procedure is painless but if you have a scan in the early part of your pregnancy you will need to have a full bladder. Don't worry about this; arrive early and drink several glasses of water.

An ultrasound scan generally takes about 5–10 minutes. You are asked beforehand to drink fluids so that your bladder is full and clearly visible to the technician. You partially undress, and then a jelly is rubbed onto your stomach and a transducer is passed over it. The transducer sends back the signals which come up on a monitor. There is no pain, just a gentle, flowing feeling.

USES OF ULTRASOUND

An ultrasound scan is used by medical staff to:
● determine the age of the fetus by taking measurements of the head and body. If done early in pregnancy, this is accurate to within one week
● measure growth, and growth retardation when clinical examination suggests something is wrong. Serial assessment, that is a number of scans over a period of time, monitors fetal growth and establishes the estimated date of delivery
● find the exact position of the baby and placenta prior to amniocentesis (see overleaf)
● locate the position of the placenta and its condition, should it become dislodged late in pregnancy
● determine if you are carrying more than one baby should alpha fetoprotein levels rise
● pick up visible abnormalities of the baby such as brain or kidney conditions
● identify any growths in the mother that might hinder delivery.

Safety considerations

Some authorities have stated that ultrasound is perfectly safe, but this is not proven. It used to be thought that X-rays of the developing embryo were safe, but it was only decades later that it was discovered that X-rays had a harmful effect on the embryo. It's fair to say, however, that all the information that we

have at the present time points to ultrasound scans being safe for mother and baby.

AFP screening

Alpha fetoprotein is a substance found in the blood of a pregnant woman in varying levels throughout pregnancy. Between 16 and 18 weeks the levels are usually low, so if your blood is examined for AFP at this time and the levels are raised, you could be carrying a baby with a neural tube defect such as spina bifida or other abnormalities of brain development. Raised levels are not, however, conclusive evidence of neural tube defect. To be certain, alpha fetoprotein must also be found in abnormal quantities in the amniotic fluid. However, as AFP may be raised with a twin pregnancy, and since it also rises as pregnancy progresses, an ultrasound scan will be taken to check for twins or to confirm your dates in case the pregnancy is more advanced. A further blood test will be taken if the checks prove negative; amniocentesis will be contemplated only if corroboration is needed.

Fetoscopy

This is the passing of a very small tube containing a light and a powerful lens into the amniotic fluid so that the developing baby can be seen directly. It is done through a small incision just above the pubic bone, with constant monitoring on ultrasound. A local anesthetic is used. A mechanical intervention of this magnitude is always considered seriously—indeed most physicians would make a determined effort to avoid it unless absolutely necessary. It is undertaken more readily at those hospitals practicing high technology births than in those that have a more natural approach.

It is carried out in week 15 of the pregnancy and is used to check for brain abnormalities, blood disorders and any visible defects such as cleft palate.

Amniocentesis

Used to detect a range of birth defects including spina bifida and mongolism or Down's syndrome (see below), this is a routine test for women over 35. It is also used if the obstetrician suspects some abnormality that cannot be detected by other tests. Though it is becoming more readily available, it is still a serious interference with your pregnancy. It involves taking a sample of the fluid surrounding the baby in the uterus. Any discarded cells floating around in the amniotic fluid will give an accurate chromosome count and denote abnormal chromosomal structure. It is also possible to find out how much oxygen and carbon dioxide is in the fluid, revealing whether the baby is getting sufficient oxygen or is at some risk.

For a woman under the age of 35, the risks of amniocentesis are statistically greater than the risks of abnormality. But if you are really concerned about the normality of your child, consult your obstetrician. Most obstetricians will agree to this if they see that you are disturbed.

Your doctor will recommend amniocentesis if you already have an abnormal child, or if there is a family history of abnormality. The sex of the baby can be determined by simply looking at some cells of the skin, so you can find out if any sex-linked disorders might have been inherited. Doctors will not do the test simply to find out the baby's sex. In cases of RH blood incompatibility, the bilirubin content of the fluid is a good indicator as to whether the baby needs an intrauterine blood transfusion (see p. 151).

HOW AMNIOCENTESIS WORKS

Amniotic fluid is swallowed by the fetus and passed out through its mouth or bladder; this fluid contains cells from the skin and other organs which provide clues to the baby's condition. Amniocentesis is the simple procedure to extract this fluid from the womb. About 75 different genetic diseases can then be subjected to chromosome analysis. The test is carried out in the hospital, generally not until 16 weeks after the last menstrual period; before then there is unlikely to be sufficient fluid in the amniotic sac and therefore cells to analyse.

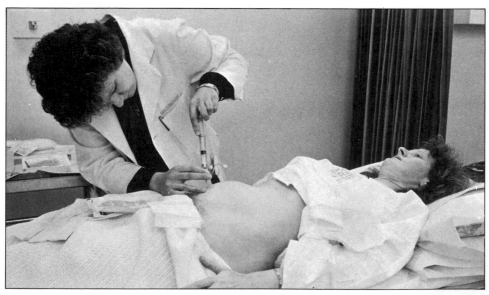

Risks of amniocentesis

With a skilled operator and the use of an ultrasonic scan to show the exact position of placenta and fetus the risk of miscarriage is minimal – 0.5 per cent in the United States, 1.2 per cent in Britain. But the decision to have amniocentesis should be weighed carefully; you should consider whether you are prepared to have your pregnancy terminated if the results give cause for concern.

Possibly the worst element of amniocentesis is the stress of waiting for the results. Also your amniotic fluid may be tested for only one abnormality, which means that a negative result may not reflect other possible problems. Tell your doctor that you want analysis and the results of all possible tests that could apply to you.

HOW THE FLUID IS EXTRACTED

After an ultrasonic scan to determine the position of the fetus and the placenta, a small area of the abdomen is treated with local anesthetic and a long hollow needle surmounted by a syringe is carefully inserted into the womb. About ½ oz of fluid is withdrawn from the amniotic sac. The fluid is then spun in a centrifuge to separate the cells shed by the baby from the rest of the liquid. The cells are cultured for 2½ to 5 weeks.

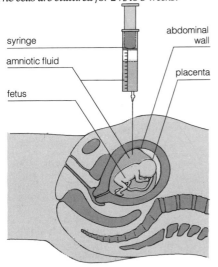

syringe

amniotic fluid

fetus

abdominal wall

placenta

REASONS FOR AMNIOCENTESIS

Amniocentesis will be offered if:
- she is over 35, when the risk of chromosomal abnormalities is greatly increased
- certain diseases run in her family such as errors of the metabolism
- she is a carrier of genetically linked disorders such as hemophilia or certain forms of muscular dystrophy, where a male child will have a 50 per cent chance of being affected
- her AFP levels are raised, suggesting spina bifida.
- a Cesarean section is planned. Tests will reveal the maturity of the baby's lungs. Immature lungs may be affected by respiratory distress syndrome.

DOWN'S SYNDROME OR MONGOLISM

This is a result of a chromosomal abnormality in the baby. In most cases an extra chromosome occurring before or immediately after fertilization gives the fetus 47 chromosomes in each cell instead of the normal 46 (see p. 28). The exact cause is unknown but maternal age is an important factor, the risk of having a Down's syndrome baby rising sharply after the age of 35.

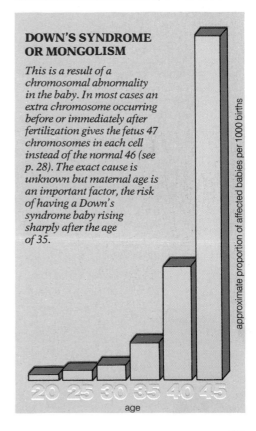

approximate proportion of affected babies per 1000 births

20 25 30 35 40 45

age

5 The growing baby

You can't see your baby growing inside you, but a great deal is now known about the incredible changes that are taking place. The sequence of developmental stages can be roughly divided into three parts or trimesters of around 12 weeks each. By the end of the first trimester, the fetus is recognizably human although only 3 in long. The second trimester is a period of rapid growth, and during the third trimester, the baby elongates and starts to accumulate fat.

LIFE SUPPORT SYSTEMS

The most crucial factor in the successful growth and development of your baby is a healthy placenta which forms the vital link between your body and your baby's. The placenta is the organ which allows your baby to lean on you and your body functions for its health and well-being. It also acts as a waste disposal unit and cleanses the baby's body of unwanted waste materials. It does so through its unique structure which allows the intermingling of your blood with your baby's blood. It is convenient to think of the mature placenta as a blood-filled space, bounded on one side by a maternal surface and on the other side by a fetal surface.

WHAT THE PLACENTA DOES
- Allows oxygen, nutrients and protective antibodies to be passed from mother to baby
- produces essential pregnancy hormones
- passes the baby's waste products to the mother for disposal.

WHAT THE AMNIOTIC FLUID DOES
- Supports the fetus while it moves freely thus exercising its muscles
- maintains a constant temperature
- acts as a cushion to protect the baby if the uterus receives a blow
- exerts a constant outward pressure on the uterus so the baby has room to grow
- in labor forms a wedge protecting the baby's head while assisting in the dilation of the cervix
- receives substances excreted by the fetus in its urine.

Amniotic fluid

From week 4 or 5, amniotic fluid fills the amniotic space which is formed by the bag of membranes enclosing the developing embryo. By week 12 the fetus is swallowing the fluid, which is absorbed through its intestines into its bloodstream. From there it passes through the umbilical cord and placenta to the mother's bloodstream (see opposite). Some fluid continues to circulate like this throughout pregnancy, but by early in the second trimester the fetus begins to use its own kidneys and urinate.

The membranes

These are two thin, papery sheets, the amnion and the chorion, which line the uterus and form the bag of waters inside which the baby develops.

BABY'S LIFE SUPPORT SYSTEM

The amniotic space and the placenta make up the baby's life support system. The amniotic space has developed deep inside the blastocyst, which was formed by the fertilized ovum. It therefore contains traces of cells which bear the sex of the embryo and the blueprint of its genetic make-up (see p. 28). The space is surrounded by the membranes and it contains the amniotic fluid or "liquor".

The placenta is joined to the baby by the umbilical cord. This cord is made up of three intertwined blood vessels. Two carry blood from the baby to the placenta for cleansing and purification. One carries oxygenated blood and nutrients to the baby. The cord is surrounded first by a jelly-like substance (Wharton's jelly), then by a membrane. The placenta itself is firmly rooted to the wall of the uterus.

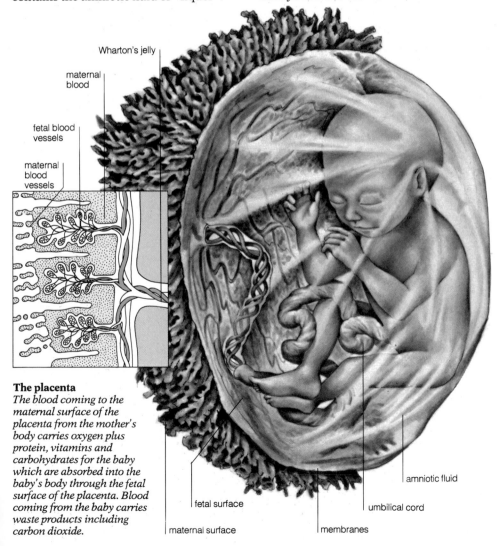

Wharton's jelly

maternal blood

fetal blood vessels

maternal blood vessels

The placenta
The blood coming to the maternal surface of the placenta from the mother's body carries oxygen plus protein, vitamins and carbohydrates for the baby which are absorbed into the baby's body through the fetal surface of the placenta. Blood coming from the baby carries waste products including carbon dioxide.

fetal surface

maternal surface

amniotic fluid

umbilical cord

membranes

71

1st Trimester

By the end of the first trimester, the systems of the fetus' body are already well developed, with many organs more or less complete. Nerves and muscles are working, and reflexes are becoming established. The heart pumps about 60 pints of blood through its circulatory system each day. Your baby can move spontaneously, although you are not aware of these movements.

The Development of the Embryo
Between weeks 5 and 7, the embryo, though still small, develops physically at a rapid rate. By week 7 the intestines are formed and the limb buds are visible. The embryo is starting to look recognizably human. The small silhouettes represent the approximate size of the embryo.

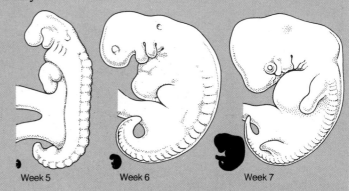

Week 5   Week 6   Week 7

WEEK 5
The embryo is quite easy to see with the naked eye. The spinal column is beginning to develop. The foundations of the brain and the spinal cord are appearing.
Length: ⅛ in

WEEK 6
The head begins to form, followed by the chest and abdomen. The heart, which is only a single tube, is beating. Blood cells are made and are circulating with each heartbeat. Blood vessels in the umbilical cord to the placenta are forming, strengthening the link between mother and baby. There are small depressions where the eyes will develop and the beginnings of a mouth. The lower jaw is visible. There are arm and leg buds.
Length: ¼ in

WEEK 7
Indentations that will form the fingers and toes are visible. The intestines are almost completely formed. The lungs are formed but they are still solid. There is dramatic development in the head. The inner parts of the ears are developing and so are the eyes. There are holes for the nostrils. Bone cells appear in what has thus far been cartilage bone. This marks the change from embryo to fetus.
Length: ¾ in

WEEK 8
All the internal organs are in place. The major joints of the shoulders, elbows, hips and knees are obvious. The spine can move. The genital organs are visible, though the fetus still looks fishlike.
Length: 1 in

WEEK 9
The mouth begins to develop and the nose is there now. The most rapidly growing parts are the limbs, hands and feet. The hearing mechanism in the ear has developed. Although you are unable to feel it, your baby is moving around quite a lot.
Length: 1 1/16 in
Weight: 1/16 oz

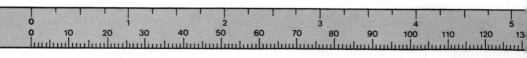

WEEK 10

The external parts of the ears are beginning to grow and the eyes are well formed. The head is still large compared to the rest of the body and its development is pronounced. The fingers and toes are distinguishable, but joined by webs of skin.
Length: 1¾ in
Weight: ⅛ oz

WEEK 11

The ovaries and testicles are formed, as are the external genital organs. The heart pumps blood to all parts of the body. By the end of week 11 all the internal organs are fully formed and functioning. Only in rare cases now will these organs be harmed by infections, chemicals or drugs.
Length: 2$\frac{3}{16}$ in
Weight: $\frac{5}{16}$ oz

WEEK 12

Closed eyelids are distinguishable as the face becomes properly formed. Muscles are starting to grow on the body which makes the limb movements more pronounced. Brain and muscles co-ordinate. Joints contract, toes will curl and it sucks. The fingers and toes are fully formed and have nails. Your baby can swallow and takes in the amniotic fluid.
Length: 3 in
Weight: ⅝ oz

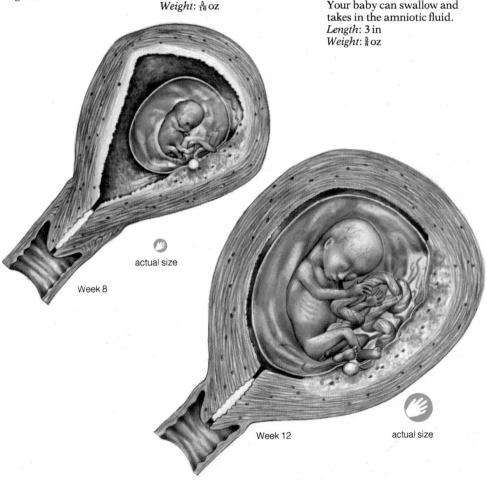

actual size

Week 8

Week 12

actual size

2nd Trimester

The middle third of pregnancy is the period in which you will feel the first fetal movements, from about week 18 onwards. Your baby is also starting to look like a real person with hair, even eyelashes, and to behave like one when it starts to suck its thumb. During this time you will become noticeably pregnant.

WEEK 13
Your baby is completely formed. During the rest of the pregnancy it simply grows to size, so that by the time it is born its vital organs have matured to make it capable of independent life.
Length: 3½ in
Weight: 1 oz

WEEK 14
The increase in weight is pronounced. All the major muscles respond to stimulation from the brain. The arms can bend from the wrist and elbow; the fingers can curl and make fists. The heart can be heard with an ultrasonic device.
Length: 4 in
Weight: 2¼ oz

WEEK 16
The limbs and joints are fully formed and the muscles are getting stronger. Movement is vigorous, though rarely felt at this stage in a first pregnancy. There is a growth of fine hair (lanugo) all over the body and eyebrows and lashes start to grow.
Length: 6 in
Weight: 4¾ oz

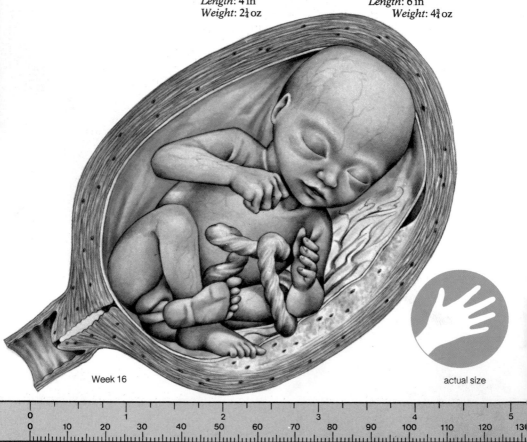

Week 16

actual size

0		1		2		3		4		5
0	10	20	30	40	50	60	70	80	90	100	110	120	130

WEEK 20

Your baby is growing very fast. The teeth are forming in the jawbone and hair is growing on the head.The muscles are increasing in strength. Movement is more vigorous and you should feel them by now. They are light flutters rather like bubbles bursting against your abdomen.

Length: 10 in
Weight: 12 oz

WEEK 24

The baby intermittently sucks its thumb and it can cough and hiccup. It hasn't yet laid down fat stores and is still thin.

Length: 13 in
Weight: 1¼ lb

WEEK 28

The head is now more in proportion to the body. Fat stores are beginning to accumulate. The body is covered in thick grease (vernix) which prevents the skin from becoming soggy from immersion in the amniotic fluid. The lungs are reaching maturity and the baby could breathe if it were born.

Length: 14½ in
Weight: 2 lb

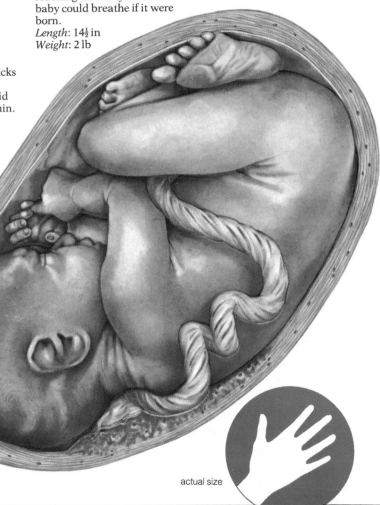

Week 28

actual size

3rd Trimester

After week 28 the baby is considered viable by the law, that is, it is capable of sustaining independent life. If born during the third trimester it might have breathing problems and difficulty keeping itself warm but with modern special care facilities it has a good chance of survival.

WEEK 32
Your baby's proportions are as you would expect them to be at birth. It is much stronger and in over 90 per cent of cases it lies with its head down towards your pelvis. Its movements are now very vigorous and clearly discernible.
Length: 16 in
Weight: 3½ lb

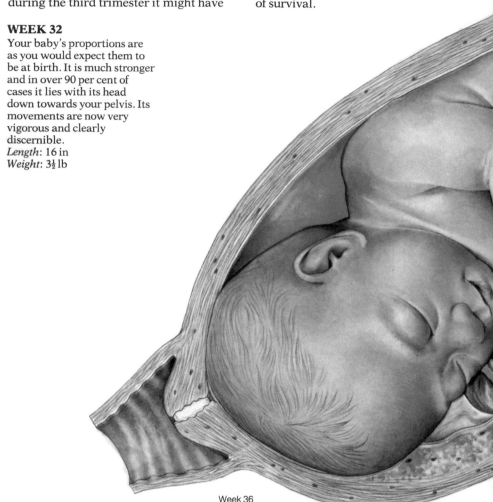

Week 36

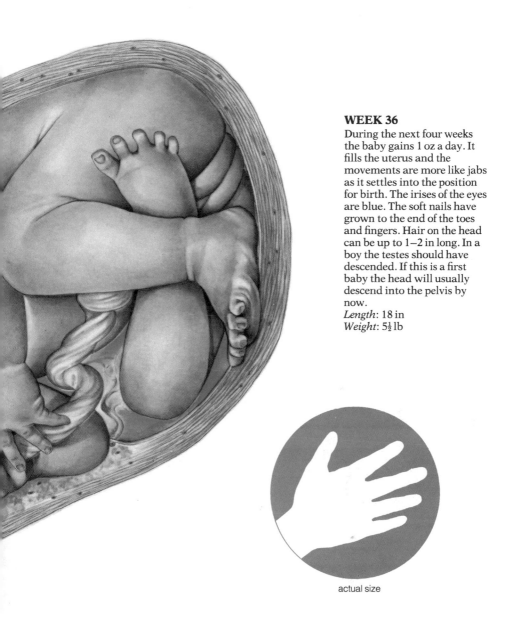

WEEK 36

During the next four weeks the baby gains 1 oz a day. It fills the uterus and the movements are more like jabs as it settles into the position for birth. The irises of the eyes are blue. The soft nails have grown to the end of the toes and fingers. Hair on the head can be up to 1–2 in long. In a boy the testes should have descended. If this is a first baby the head will usually descend into the pelvis by now.
Length: 18 in
Weight: 5½ lb

actual size

6   7   8   9   10   11
150 160 170 180 190 200 210 220 230 240 250 260 270 280

Term

Forty weeks after the first day of your last menstrual period your baby is ready to be born, though babies rarely arrive on the estimated day of delivery (see p. 37). With second and subsequent babies, the head engages in the bony pelvic opening about one week before the birth or in some cases not until labor has started.

WEEK 40
The vernix has decreased so that there are only remnants in the skin folds – around the neck, armpits and groin. The nails on the fingers are long and will need cutting shortly after birth. When the baby is awake its eyes are open and it can discern light. Most of the lanugo has gone.
Length: 20 in
Weight: 7½ lb

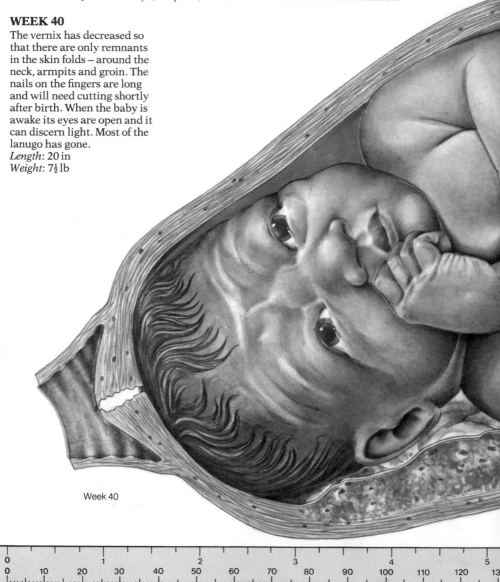

Week 40

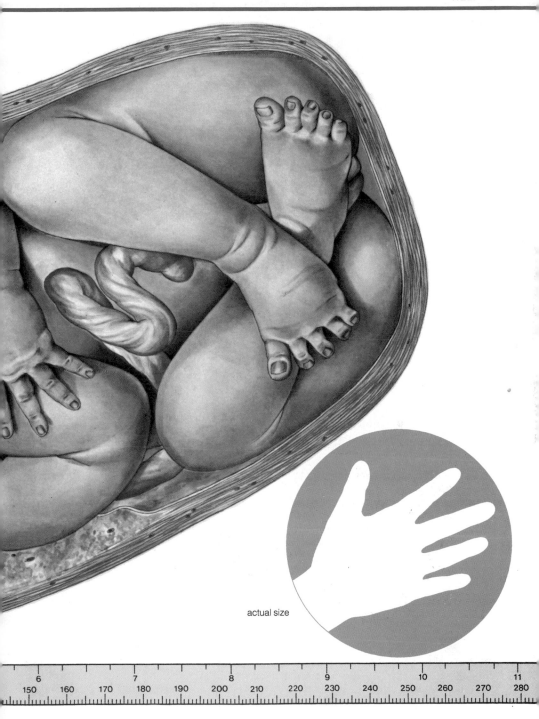

actual size

6 Physical changes

Nearly all the changes in your body that you can see and feel, such as enlargement of the breasts, deepening pigmentation of the skin, and slight breathlessness on exertion, are due in one way or another to the increased production of a range of female and pregnancy hormones. Early in pregnancy your ovaries are responsible for the main output, but very quickly the maternal supply begins to be overtaken by that from the placenta. The output of hormones is colossal. For instance, at any time during an average menstrual cycle, the maximum daily output of one key hormone, progesterone, would be a few milligrams a day; towards the end of pregnancy this rises to as much as 250mg a day. While progesterone output increases 50–60 times, that of another key hormone, estrogen, increases 20–30 times. All the hormones cause changes to take place in your body's structure and processes so that it can support and nourish your developing baby. No organ escapes the effects of these biochemical alterations.

MENSTRUAL CYCLE

The first deviation from normal hormonal patterns occurs very early in pregnancy. The menstrual cycle begins when a hormone (follicle-stimulating hormone – FSH) from the pituitary gland stimulates the development of an egg (ovum) in a follicle inside one of the ovaries (see p. 30). In a 28-day menstrual cycle (see p. 27), ovulation occurs around day 14 when the follicle bursts, discharging the ovum, which starts to move down the Fallopian tube towards the uterus. It is helped by "fingers" at the end of the Fallopian tube which direct it on its way. Also at this time, the lining of the uterus (endometrium) begins to thicken and the mucus at the neck of the uterus (cervix) becomes thinner so that the sperm can gain an easier entry. If the ovum is not fertilized, at around day 24 the decaying follicle (corpus luteum) begins to wither, and further hormonal changes result in shedding of the endometrium on day 28 and bleeding on day 1 of the next cycle.

When pregnancy occurs, fertilization happens around day 14 of the cycle, then implantation of the fertilized ovum in the uterine wall begins some seven days after that, around day 21. There are, therefore, three or four days between implantation and the usual regression of the corpus luteum. The body has only this short interval in which to stop the regression and suppress menstruation. This is probably achieved by a powerful hormone called human chorionic gonadotrophin (HCG), which is produced by the fertilized ovum and whose immediate function is thought to be the maintenance of both a healthy corpus luteum and the levels of estrogen and progesterone coming from the ovaries. In this way, the mother's body and the developing embryo, which at this stage is only a minute ball of cells (see p. 30), co-operate to prevent menstruation and keep the pregnancy intact.

Some pregnant women's hormonal levels are not sufficiently increased to prevent breakthrough bleeding at the time of their first missed period and, for a few, slight breakthrough bleeding may occur at the time when the second and even third missed periods were due. In this case the blood comes from the endometrium, not the fertilized ovum, and bleeding does not harm the baby. However, if hormonal levels are too low, a miscarriage will almost certainly occur (see p. 148).

The placenta

In order to become implanted, part of the fertilized ovum puts out microscopic fingerlike protrusions (chorionic villi), which embed themselves in the wall of the uterus. These protrusions become the placenta, which supplies food and oxygen to the baby and carries waste from it. Well within the first trimester, the placenta has developed into an efficient chemical factory, producing an ever-increasing supply of female and pregnancy hormones with two specific functions. First, these hormones alter the mother's body so that pregnancy can be maintained and lactation prepared for. Second, they ensure that the reproductive organs are in a healthy state, and that the placenta functions efficiently, so keeping the baby well nourished and alive.

28-DAY MENSTRUAL CYCLE

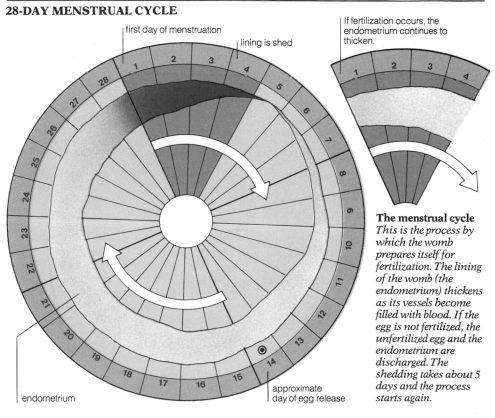

first day of menstruation

lining is shed

If fertilization occurs, the endometrium continues to thicken.

endometrium

approximate day of egg release

The menstrual cycle
This is the process by which the womb prepares itself for fertilization. The lining of the womb (the endometrium) thickens as its vessels become filled with blood. If the egg is not fertilized, the unfertilized egg and the endometrium are discharged. The shedding takes about 5 days and the process starts again.

HORMONES OF PREGNANCY

Name	Action	Effect on mother and baby
Human chorionic gonadotrophin (HCG)	Produced by the chorionic villi, causes the ovary to produce more progesterone (see below), thus suppressing menstruation and sustaining the pregnancy. Reaches a peak of production around the 70th day and then falls to a constant value for the rest of the pregnancy. Maintains the function of the ovaries until the placenta takes over.	High levels in the bloodstream parallel the time when women normally suffer from nausea in pregnancy (see p. 35), could be associated with morning sickness. Detection of this hormone in urine is a reliable pregnancy test (see p. 36).
Human placental lactogen (HPL)	Produced by the placenta, it is essential to normal milk production. Its presence is used as a test to indicate the efficiency of the placenta in late pregnancy.	Enlarges the breasts and causes secretion of colostrum from about the fifth month. Low levels indicate the placenta may not be functioning well enough to nourish the baby.
Relaxin	Probably produced by the placenta and ovary. In animal experiments, it was found to soften the uterine cervix. Relaxes the pelvic joints.	May have an effect of relaxing the ligaments and joints.
Estrogens	Produced in the placenta using starter substances from the mother's and the baby's adrenal glands.	Affects all aspects of pregnancy. It is particularly important in maintaining the health of the genital tract, the reproductive organs and the breasts.
Progesterone	Produced in the same way as estrogen. Sustains the pregnancy, relaxes smooth muscle.	Affects all aspects of pregnancy. Prepares the breasts for lactation. Relaxation of joints and ligaments in preparation for childbirth can affect bowel movements, causing constipation (see p. 136) and resulting in back pain (see p. 140). Raises body temperature.
Melanocyte stimulating hormone (MSH)	Higher levels than normal during pregnancy. Stimulates the skin to produce pigment.	Increase in color of the nipples, patches of brown pigmentation on the face, inner thighs and a brown line running down the centre of the abdomen (see p. 88). Some women notice none of these changes.

BREASTS

Size and shape vary from individual to individual and according to the point in the menstrual cycle. In the second half of the cycle, after ovulation day, most women experience some enlargement of their breasts. Just before menstruation, the consistency becomes rather nodular as the milk glands enlarge, the tinted areas around the nipples (areolas) become slightly bumpy as the sebaceous glands enlarge, and the nipples become sensitive. Changes in the breasts during pregnancy may be one of the earliest signs of pregnancy that you become aware of.

Most women with an average 28-day cycle will notice a definite enlargement of the breasts by week 6–8 of pregnancy, two to four weeks after their first missed period would have started. The breasts will feel firm and generally tender and have more and larger veins than usual running close to the surface of the skin. Tingling is common, as are occasional stabbing pains. The sebaceous glands on the areolas

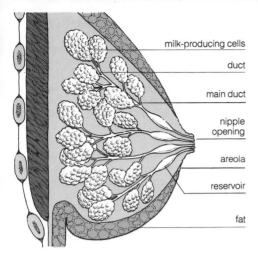

milk-producing cells

duct

main duct

nipple
opening

areola

reservoir

fat

*The cross section of the lactating breast looks
rather like a tree with many branches and leaves.*

From early pregnancy your breasts will be
making a form of milk called colostrum
(see p. 209). This may be secreted either
involuntarily or by massage (see below)
although there is nothing to worry about if
you can't express any. There shouldn't be
enough during pregnancy to cause you
embarrassment.

Most of the growth of the ducts and
increase in size and weight of the breasts
occurs in the first trimester. This is a result
of the increase in the number of milk ducts
in preparation for lactation. During these
first three months, you should be fitted for
a good bra. You will probably need one at
least two bra sizes larger. You will also
need nursing bras after the baby is born
(see p. 125). If you support the weight of
your breasts during pregnancy and
lactation they will return to the pre-
pregnant shape and firmness when you
stop breastfeeding. Some women find
their breasts are smaller after weaning, as
the original fat in the breasts has been
replaced by milk-producing ducts.
Towards the end of the first trimester you
will see one of the last changes in the
breasts, darkening of the nipples and
areolas due to a general increase in
pigmentation (see p. 88) which is another
characteristic of pregnancy.

(Montgomery's tubercles) become raised,
nodular and pink.

The breasts are composed mainly of
millions of tiny milk glands plus their
small ducts, joined together to come out at
the nipple. Although there is almost
certainly some overlap in the effect of
hormones, estrogen stimulates the growth
of the ducts while progesterone stimulates
enlargement of the glands themselves.

Expressing colostrum
*To do this during
pregnancy, hold your
elbows straight out to
the sides and with your
palms against your rib
cage, massage in
towards the nipple with
a gentle but firm
pressure.*

Flat or inverted nipples
*You can improve them by wearing breast shields
under your bra from about week 15. Wear them
for a few hours at first, building up to several
hours each day in the third trimester. They are
made of plastic or glass and they have a hole in
them through which the nipple is gently pulled by
suction. This is not painful.*

THE UTERUS

Three principal tasks are performed by the uterus during pregnancy. It is the site of implantation by the fertilized ovum, it accommodates the growing baby, and it expels the baby at term. To achieve the second of these tasks the uterus has to grow and distend, while restraining a normal tendency to contract when there is something inside it and while the outlet, the cervix, remains resistant to stretching.

Expansion

To accommodate the developing baby, placenta and surrounding fluids, the internal volume of the uterus has to expand from being a potential space to one of about 11 pints – an increase in volume of some 1000 times.

In the first half of pregnancy, the uterus gains weight quickly mainly due to an increase in the size of the muscle fibers. Each muscle cell of the uterus increases in size by as much as 50 times, initially under the stimulation of estrogen. Around mid-pregnancy this rate of growth slows down, but uterine volume then increases rapidly as the muscle fibers stretch and thin out. All this growth results in the uterus increasing its weight some 20 times, from about 2½oz to 38oz at term. The expansion is not noticeable until about week 16 when the uterus begins to rise out of the pelvis. By week 36 the top of the uterus has risen to just below the breast bone. When the baby's head engages (see p. 159), it descends again.

THE EXPANDING UTERUS
The uterus increases its volume about 1000 times in pregnancy and as it does, it crowds out the other organs. This can result in problems such as frequency of urination, heartburn, breathlessness and constipation.

diaphragm

stomach

intestines

uterus

fetus

bladder

vagina

rectum

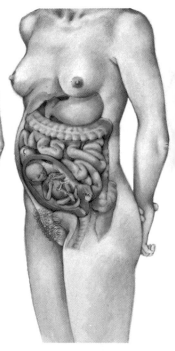

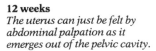

12 weeks
The uterus can just be felt by abdominal palpation as it emerges out of the pelvic cavity.

16 weeks
The uterus is expanding quickly, your waist disappears and you are noticeably pregnant.

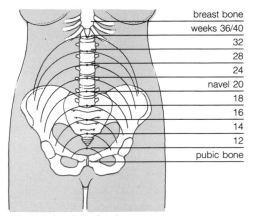

breast bone
weeks 36/40
32
28
24
navel 20
18
16
14
12
pubic bone

The height of the fundus
This can be determined by abdominal palpation or by measuring in centimeters from the pubic bone. This measurement is used as a guide to the duration of your pregnancy.

Contractions

One of the normal characteristics of uterine muscle is that it undergoes contractions which are hardly ever felt. All the way through pregnancy the uterus contracts in a weak, short-lived way that you may or may not notice, although if you put a hand on your abdomen you can feel the muscle going tight and hard. These slight, painless movements are called Braxton Hicks contractions and occur about every 20 minutes throughout pregnancy. They are important in ensuring a good blood circulation through the uterus; they also help uterine growth. You probably won't notice Braxton Hicks contractions until the last month of your pregnancy. They can become quite strong and may be mistaken for labor. This is called "false labor" (see p. 161).

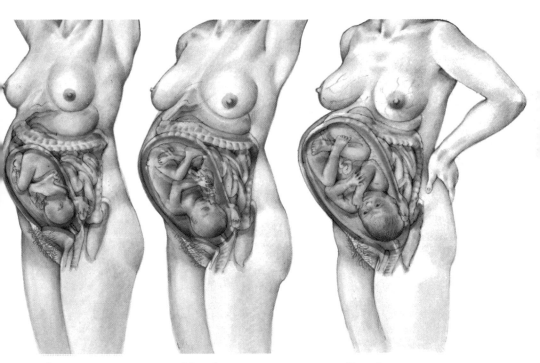

28 weeks
The skin on your abdomen will start to stretch and the upward pressure may lead to indigestion.

36 weeks
The uterus is now putting pressure on your rib cage and you may feel jabbing pain there.

40 weeks
The baby's head will engage in the pelvic cavity and put pressure on the groin and pelvis.

Up until weeks 12 to 14, the developing baby can quite easily be accommodated in the space within the growing uterus, but after this time the junction of the uterus and the top of the cervix begins to smooth out, giving the baby more space. This part is called the lower segment of the uterus. It is essential that the smoothing out of this lower segment doesn't allow the cervix to dilate before the baby is ready to be born.

While the upper half of the cervix is muscular and stretchy, the lower half contains a strong, tight band of fibrous tissue. Although this band softens during pregnancy, especially in the last weeks, to prepare for the birth, its resistance to dilation is usually sufficient to withstand Braxton Hicks contractions. During labor, it is the upper segment of the uterus that contracts to push the baby out.

VAGINA

Early in pregnancy, the vaginal tissues also change so that the vagina will dilate more easily for the birth. The muscle cells enlarge and the mucus membranes of the lining thicken. One side effect of this is an increase in vaginal secretions (see p. 142) which may mean you need light sanitary pads for comfort. If the secretion has an offensive smell or makes you sore, tell your doctor and never douche during pregnancy. One other result of this increased lubrication and swelling of the vagina may be an increase in sexual pleasure. This, however, differs from woman to woman and will vary throughout the pregnancy (see p. 94).

VITAL FUNCTIONS

Your body will react to the hormonal stimulation of pregnancy by widespread changes in the important circulatory, respiratory and urinary systems. It used to be thought that the relationship between the mother and embryo was simply that of host and parasite but we now know that it is much more complex. From the earliest days, in response to diversified and raised hormonal output, the mother continually anticipates the needs of her baby: by changes in her vital functions, she precedes the baby's demands.

Blood

During pregnancy , the volume of blood increases by about 45 per cent above non-pregnant levels to 14 pints. The volume gradually increases from about week 10, reaching a plateau in the third trimester. The extra blood is required by the uterus, which takes about 25 per cent; the breasts; and other vital organs – even the gums receive an increase in their blood supply (see p. 89). The increase in the liquid part of the blood (plasma) is proportionately greater than that of the red cells. If the red cells become too diluted, this will show up in prenatal blood tests as a fall in the hemoglobin concentration; this is known as physiological anemia. It is not the same thing as iron-deficiency anemia (see p. 61). In a normal pregnant woman, the number of red blood cells multiplies steadily, particularly if you include a lot of iron in your diet.

Another effect of the increase of fluids circulating in the body is a lowering of the sodium concentration, which is why, contrary to usual dietary advice, you shouldn't restrict your salt intake during pregnancy (see p. 103) unless you have serious fluid retention.

Heart

With more fluids to push around the body, the heart has extra work to do. By the end of the second trimester it has increased its workload by 40 per cent. It enlarges to accommodate this extra work and your pulse rate is raised 10–15 beats per minute during pregnancy. Much of the circulation increase is directed to the uterus. Blood flow to the kidneys also increases. The quantity of blood flowing through your skin goes up too, and this is why your skin appears pinker, is warmer and sweats more. During the third trimester, the uterus may press on the large vein in the abdomen if you lie on your back. This causes blood pressure to fall and may make you feel dizzy and faint so turn on your side when resting.

Lungs

To keep the extra blood well supplied with oxygen, the lungs have to work harder too. If you get plenty of fresh air and exercise, blood supply to the lungs will be improved. During the third trimester, particularly if you have a multiple pregnancy or are very large, the uterus will begin to crowd the lungs out. You may feel uncomfortable, and find yourself having to take deep breaths. Sitting up straight helps, even in bed.

Kidneys

Your kidneys have to filter and clean 45 per cent more blood than they did before. As a result, all renal function becomes more efficient, the body getting rid of waste products like urea and uric acid faster than before. But the kidneys don't distinguish between waste products and nutrients, so glucose is also quickly cleared from the blood, together with minerals and vitamins – for instance, water-soluble vitamin C, plus folic acid, which is excreted at four or five times the usual rate. This is one of the reasons for making sure your general nutrition, and particularly your vitamin and mineral intake, is maintained during pregnancy, and why you may need folic acid supplements (see p. 103).

In addition to the greater amount of urine to be got rid of, the contracting uterus irritates the neighboring bladder, so that you will probably find you need to pass urine more frequently than usual. This is one of the earliest signs of pregnancy (see p. 35). Even though this is annoying, don't restrict your fluid intake in an attempt to control it.

Joints

Bands of tough and inflexible fibrous tissue called ligaments surround and connect joints, supporting and strengthening them and keeping them stable. With the advent of pregnancy, and the secretion of certain hormones, these ligaments, especially in the pelvis, begin to soften and become more flexible. This is in preparation for labor when most of the joints in the pelvis can give and mold to allow your baby a smooth passage to the outside world. The joints mainly affected are the sacroiliac joint in the lower back, plus the junction of the pubic bones which lies at the front, the symphysis pubis.

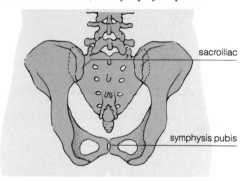

Sacroiliac joint
This joint is located at the top of the buttocks.

After about week 16, the weight of the growing baby pushing down in the pelvis can tip the pelvic brim forward. This changed angle, together with the ever-growing weight that is being carried, puts strain on the muscles and ligaments surrounding the lower spine, which is one reason for backache. You can counter the forward tilt with good posture and by doing pelvic tilt exercises (see p. 118).

The elasticity of all the ligaments during pregnancy means they are more liable to be stretched, and therefore ache, particularly in the lower back, legs and feet. Good posture (see p. 108), exercise, shoes with some support and massage (see p. 133) can do a lot to counteract discomfort (see pp. 136–143).

SKIN

Though some women do glow with good health during pregnancy, there are some changes to the skin that are not so flattering. They usually, however, disappear shortly after the birth of the baby.

Pigmentation

Some degree of darkening is a universal characteristic of pregnancy, although its depth varies according to skin color. Blondes, redheads, and even brunettes who have pale skins may see little change, whereas olive-skinned women may find that their whole skin goes several shades darker, and areas like the nipples, areolas, abdomen, and genital region remain dark brown for the rest of their lives.

Pigmentation of the nipples and areolas and a dark line down the centre of the abdomen, called the linea nigra, usually make their appearance around week 14. The linea nigra can be up to ½in wide and stretches from the pubic hair to the navel, or even up to the breast bone. The navel tends to darken, and by the third trimester it flattens out, being completely flat by 40 weeks. It returns to normal after delivery. The linea nigra also begins to fade shortly after delivery, but may take several months to disappear completely, or remain as a shadow.

Any brown birthmarks, moles, freckles, or recent scars, particularly on the abdomen, may darken during pregnancy, the effect becoming more obvious after exposure to sunlight, but they will probably return to normal shortly after delivery. Blotchy and irregular brown patches (chloasma) sometimes appear and are made worse by sunlight (see p. 126). They usually begin to fade shortly after delivery and may disappear completely in a few months.

Texture

It's impossible to anticipate whether your skin, particularly on your face, will become drier or oilier, improve or get worse during pregnancy. High levels of hormones have several effects on skin, as does the greater amount of blood circulating to it. Oiliness results from the action of progesterone, which encourages the secretion of sebum. Pimples can appear unexpectedly (see p. 127) because of fluctuating hormone levels, not just on the face, but the back too. Increased fluid retention can fill out lines or cause unwelcome puffiness (see p. 127), depending on your face shape. However, these changes are all normal and will disappear after your baby is born.

Stretch marks

These occur in the skin under several different conditions. The first is in adolescence when we grow quickly. The second is whenever we put on a large amount of weight in a short time, and the third is during pregnancy. The underlying cause is always the same – tearing of collagen bundles. Collagen is the "skeleton" of the skin; its network of elastic bundles allows the skin to stretch with movement or with a change in size or shape.

The marks in pregnancy are due to the high level of sex hormones that are circulating in the blood. One of the effects of these hormones is to break down and remove protein from the skin thereby disrupting the collagen bundles and making the skin thin and papery. It appears delicate and stretchy in certain areas. The stretchmarks that occur when we put on a lot of weight result when the collagen bundles are stretched to the point of breaking by the fat, which is laid down underneath the skin.

During pregnancy, these marks appear on the breasts, the abdomen, and also on the thighs and buttocks. They will remain pinkish throughout pregnancy, but after delivery they shrink and become a silvery color. Stretchmarks in black women may be quite noticeable because their color is in contrast to the rest of their skin.

HAIR AND NAILS

These are both made from the same substance – keratin – and you may notice dramatic changes to your hair (see also p. 126) and finger nails during pregnancy.

Hair changes

Pregnancy can have an unpredictable and quite dramatic effect on hair. Curls may straighten out or straight hair become curly, and these changes can remain after your baby is born. Some women's hair becomes luxurious and shiny; others, lifeless or greasy. Even body hair may become more or less apparent.

Most women's hair becomes more oily, particularly towards the end of the pregnancy, due to the very high levels of progesterone in the blood, which stimulate the sebaceous glands on the scalp. Dry hair may benefit from this change, though it can make hair lank. If you've always had normal hair, you may find any change difficult to live with because your hair won't be as predictable as it was before. Because of this unpredictability pregnancy is not a good time to dye your hair or have a permanent.

One reason hair may become progressively thicker is that hormonal changes cause more than 90 per cent of the hair on your head to be thrown simultaneously into a growing phase (normally only 90 per cent are growing and the remainder resting). Therefore, during pregnancy, your hair should be thicker and stronger, although this will not apply to every woman.

Soon after birth the hair that you would normally lose, but didn't because of your pregnancy, will be lost in large amounts, making way for the new. Hair loss can go on for anything up to 18 months and, if replacement is too slow, the hair becomes thinner and thinner. This can be alarming, but no woman has gone bald simply as a result of pregnancy, so be assured that your hair will eventually recover.

Body and facial hair go into a growing phase, too, and may increase in quantity and strength. Women with dark skins, in whom pregnancy causes a greatly increased amount of pigmentation, may find that their body and facial hair darken. In some cases this hair does not return to its former color.

Nail changes

Splitting and breaking of nails is another problem that some women notice in pregnancy. It can be irritating, but rubber gloves and hand lotion can protect the nail area. They will return to normal after delivery, although those who have stronger, shinier nails in pregnancy may suffer brittleness after delivery.

TEETH AND GUMS

It used to be said that a baby absorbed the calcium from its mother's teeth and therefore women were more susceptible to decay during pregnancy than normal. This is not so, as there is no way of extracting calcium from the teeth. However, the high levels of progesterone that are produced during pregnancy will make the margins of the gums around the teeth soft and spongy, predisposing them to infection (see p. 138). It is therefore essential that you are meticulous about oral hygiene, making sure that you brush your teeth after every meal and particularly after eating anything sweet. Make an appointment to see your dentist as soon as you know you are pregnant and ask him if you should have any special care. He may suggest hardening the gum margins or using dental floss for thorough cleaning between the teeth. Keep up your regular check-ups throughout pregnancy and lactation. Remember to tell your dentist that you are pregnant, as you should avoid X-rays. The best way to avoid problems with teeth and gums is through a diet rich in calcium and vitamins and avoiding the sugary foods that lead to tooth decay.

7 Emotional changes

Psychologically speaking, your main task during the nine months of pregnancy is to incorporate your new baby into your long-term planning, your future, your feelings and your lifestyle. Though there are similar challenges for men and women, you can be affected differently. Any emotional turmoil you feel is a positive force to guide you through your adjustment to becoming a mother or father. Having gone through it, there's a good chance that you'll be emotionally well prepared for your new baby. The fact that you may have second thoughts doesn't mean that you've made a mistake. It would be wrong to think that having a baby is all fun. The best thing you can do for yourself is to be open about your feelings. If you express them to one another honestly, you will clarify your thinking and prepare the basis for a constant exchange throughout the pregnancy.

SELF-IMAGE

The size and shape of your body may make you feel strange about yourself; you may even worry about becoming fat and unattractive. Try to be positive about your shape. Look for the beauty in the fullness of your breasts and the curve of your abdomen; a pregnant woman is beautiful in her own way. For both men and women, a pregnant body is extremely sensuous. Your image of yourself in this condition is important. The self-confidence that comes with feeling proud of your shape and your fertility will make you more positive about your condition. Take a general interest in looking good (see p. 122) and being healthy (see p. 99) and fit (see pp. 108–121).

How hormones affect your mood

Mood changes are largely a reflection of the tremendous changes in your internal hormonal secretions. In a way you're hardly in control of them, so there's no reason why you should feel guilty or ashamed if you behave differently towards people; they should not judge you too harshly if, for example, you snap at them when previously you were less quick to show temper. Due to this hormonal upheaval, nearly all pregnant women are emotionally labile and given to swinging moods, extreme reactions to minor events, bouts of crying and feeling unsure and panicky. Even in the most positive of pregnancies you're going to feel some depression, fear and confusion. Once you know that it's normal to feel low every now and then in pregnancy, you'll feel better about it and your moods will pass more quickly. Try not to be too analytical; react to the next thing that comes along, which may lift you out of your bad mood.

The way to see yourself and your roundness is as something that is ripening and creating.

90

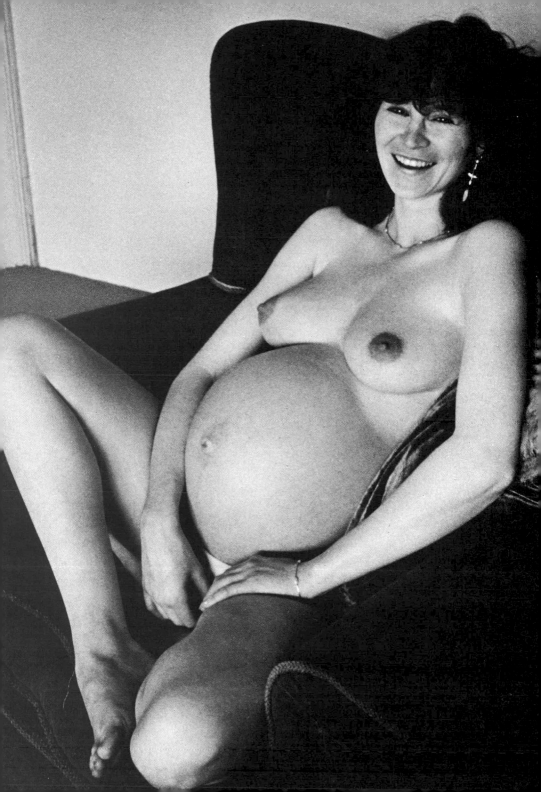

FEELINGS ABOUT YOUR PARTNER

There are going to be many ups and downs for you and your partner to cope with during pregnancy. Be prepared for them and give them time and patience. If you're in a good partnership, one of the things that you'll almost certainly feel is that the pregnancy cements your relationship. This strengthening of your bonds may be a little claustrophobic at first until you get used to it. It might help if you agree from the very beginning that you will talk about things relating to the pregnancy in an open way and that you will not interpret your partner's comments as rejection or unkindness. During this time it's quite common for couples to make unusual demands on each other as a test of loyalty and devotion. Be realistic about small grievances and be quick to point them out and explain them to each other. The reality of approaching parenthood can sometimes cause tension, but this can usually be defused if you decide to be frank with each other. Friction and conflict seem to diminish when each partner is prepared to be generous.

You'll certainly start evaluating each other in the light of your new roles. You may have always had an image of the kind of parent you would want your mate to be, and you'll try to see how he or she measures up to your fantasy. Don't be too hard in your evaluation: remember, you are evaluating yourself in the same way. This will make you sympathetic as to how your mate will feel about being judged all the time.

The special bond of pregnancy can bring you closer together in a loving relationship.

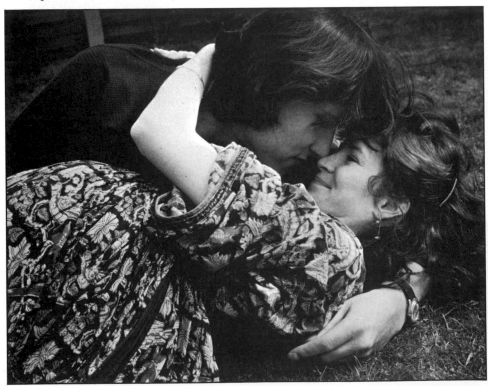

BEING AN INVOLVED FATHER

Every father needs to take an active rather than a passive role in a basic life event such as the birth of his child. You need to feel that you're contributing something too and even better that you're doing something important together.

Becoming a father doesn't start with the birth of your child: get involved with your partner's pregnancy from the beginning. Nearly all women are helped by the presence of their partner for the first prenatal visit, for example.

As a prospective father, you may be wondering how you can help your partner through her pregnancy while making sure that your own needs are met, but you have to be prepared for your life to be disrupted to some extent. The golden rule is to be observant of your partner's needs, to assist in her care, and to be closely linked with everything that's happening to her. Fatherhood always involves hard work, a lot of responsibility and a considerable amount of time but will repay you with immeasurable joy, satisfaction and happiness. During pregnancy, the delivery and after the birth, your partner will be depending on you for courage and support. If she doesn't get them from you she will feel alone.

It's not uncommon for a father-to-be to discover feelings of jealousy during a first pregnancy. You may feel neglected if your partner seems more ready to share information about her pregnancy with women friends rather than you. If you find that you are trying to minimize her requests, her problems and needs, take a look at yourself. Make a special effort to be reasonable, and listen, sympathize and encourage. She will almost certainly return your gifts, which means acceptance of you as both lover and now the father of the child.

The interdependence on one another is not easy in practice; certain traditions of bringing up boys don't facilitate it. The strong, silent loner doesn't easily make an involved loving father. It's easier to learn from a good parent who acts as an example, but you may have to educate yourself into fatherhood by devising your own way of learning.

It may make you feel better to know that mothers and fathers start off more or less equally ignorant about babies and small children. Mothers do eventually learn something out of necessity and trial and error. Unless you're involved, you'll not even be that lucky. It's a tragedy to miss out on the care of your child and instead remain a kind of stranger. Also remember that there's no one right or wrong way to be a parent, but you do have to be ready to grow just as your child is growing – in caring, in admitting mistakes, and in making time available among your family members – all these things will help to make you a better father.

SPECIAL ANXIETIES

Nearly every prospective parent, but particularly a mother, is beset by anxieties about the baby, especially in the last trimester. The immediacy of delivery and having a new baby nurtures natural anxieties about whether the baby will have any kind of abnormality, whether you will be a capable parent, whether you will do something silly like dropping the baby and whether you will be able to cope with the day-to-day care in the first weeks. All of these feelings are quite natural and most women harbor them. If you know that they are going to occur and are normal and natural, this will help to defuse your anxiety.

Dreams in particular can be disturbing. You may dream of mistreating your baby or not caring for it properly. You may dream of losing the baby or that it may be stillborn. Your dreams represent a perfectly legitimate fear in both these respects; fear that you have at the back of your mind, but during your waking hours are not prepared to face. Dreams are the way of bringing these feelings to the surface and thereby getting rid of them. Think of your dreams as a release to your anxieties. The fact that you may dream about harming your baby doesn't mean that you really want to or ever would; it's a healthy symptom of wanting to do the best for your baby.

Every pregnant woman at some stage worries about something being wrong or going wrong with the baby. Dreaming about losing the baby or about having a stillbirth has little foundation in reality. It's more likely to do with figuratively losing the baby from your uterus. Dreams about the baby dying are part of your understandable concern for your baby's

well-being. Even though I knew that dreams of this kind were perfectly natural, I still worried about having them. One way of dealing with them was to try to put them out of my head upon waking and getting on with some pleasurable aspect of preparing for the baby's arrival.

All women are beset by fears of how they'll behave in labor. Will the pain be too much? Will they scream? Will the bowels or bladder empty embarrassingly? Will they lose control of themselves and act foolishly? Will they shout and do things they wish they hadn't? Such fears are normal and the chances are you'll be surprised at how calmly you behave, though most of us do something rather silly at some time during the labor and birth. It really isn't too important. And remember the nurses and doctors have seen it all before and cannot be embarrassed.

SEX IN PREGNANCY

The majority of women I have spoken to about sex and pregnancy have almost universally felt that sex was better than ever. Because of the high level of circulating hormones, a woman can become stimulated more readily and reach a high pitch of sexual excitement more quickly than in the non-pregnant state. Many parts of her body, like the breasts, nipples and genital area (see p. 86), are more sensitive because all the sexual organs become highly developed and more capable of arousal than before pregnancy occurred. Also there is the freedom from having to use contraceptive methods.

There does, however, tend to be some loss of libido during the first and third trimesters. This could be a result of increased hormonal activity at the beginning of pregnancy, causing nausea and tiredness, and of your large shape at the end. Even if you don't feel like making love, and many couples don't, explore other ways of touching and giving sexual pleasure to each other.

There seem to be no medical reasons why you should not enjoy full sexual intercourse throughout your pregnancy; the womb is completely sealed off by the mucus plug. However, a recent article in a British medical journal has pointed out that a great deal of sexual activity might make a woman more susceptible to maternal infections. The report showed that this was almost entirely confined to lower socio-economic groups and probably related to other factors including hygiene, even possibly different sexual partners. As long as you have sex only with your partner, and only when you feel like it, and as long as it isn't too athletic, sex is to be recommended throughout pregnancy, unless your doctor advises you otherwise or other factors relate to your condition (see opposite). Sex is good for your body too – orgasm exercises the uterine muscles though this can cause contractions later on in pregnancy, which die down after a few minutes. You will also become more aware of your pelvic floor muscles.

Will sex harm the baby?

There is no information suggesting that sex harms the baby. Sex cannot introduce infection to the baby because it is safely protected in a bag of fluid that completely surrounds it. Sex will not crush the baby either. The bag of fluid (amniotic sac) is an excellent cushion and once the baby is firmly attached to its mother's uterus, there is no way that intercourse can cause a miscarriage. If the baby miscarries it's for reasons other than the fact you are having sexual intercourse, as is true of the onset of labor. Labor will not start simply because of the stimulation of sex.

WHEN NOT TO HAVE SEX

● If bleeding occurs, consult your doctor immediately and refrain from further intercourse. It may not be serious (see p. 142), but your doctor has to rule out the possibility of placenta previa (see p. 144) or of miscarriage.
● If you have had a previous miscarriage (see p. 148), ask your doctor's advice. You may be advised to abstain during the early months while the pregnancy establishes itself.
● If you have a show (see p. 161) or the waters break, there is a risk of infection.

POSITIONS FOR INTERCOURSE DURING PREGNANCY

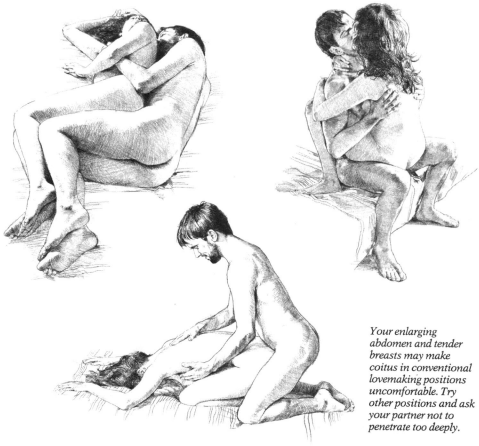

Your enlarging abdomen and tender breasts may make coitus in conventional lovemaking positions uncomfortable. Try other positions and ask your partner not to penetrate too deeply.

95

8 Health and nutrition

To ensure that your baby develops in a healthy environment, you should keep your body as fit and well nourished as you possibly can. While you don't need to devise a special diet for pregnancy, you do need to eat a good variety of the right foods – those that are rich in the essential nutrients. If you are deficient in any part of your diet, this will affect not only your health but how well you can support the pregnancy and nourish the baby. You need also to be aware of the possible harmful effects of nicotine, alcohol and drugs as they can have a detrimental effect on the growth and well-being of the baby.

WEIGHT GAIN

In pregnancy you should, for your own good and that of the baby, gain weight. These days it is believed you should gain a lot more than was thought healthy in the past. It is now known that a reasonable, not excessive, weight gain is essential. An average weight gain by women in pregnancy is around 25lb, with the most rapid gain usually between weeks 24 and 32. Your uterus, plus the baby, placenta and fluids will account for more than half of your total weight gain. You also manufacture more blood (see p. 86) and need to lay down fat early in preparation for lactation. These stores of fat remain after delivery and usually disappear gradually with breastfeeding and exercise.

In the past an alarmist attitude to too great a gain in weight was encouraged by doctors who categorized excessive weight gain as a risk factor in pregnancy. I would not want to encourage anyone to gain an excessive amount of weight, but I do feel that medical practitioners can make pregnant women unhappy with their obsessions about weight. Dieting is not a good idea in pregnancy. Eating a balanced and varied diet is. The worst effects of insufficient or variable food intake would occur in the early days and during the last trimester when the baby's brain is developing and maturing.

A recent British study showed that when there were discrepancies between mothers' calorie, vitamin and mineral intakes and current recommended levels, there was a higher incidence of low-birthweight babies amongst those women who ate less well. On the other hand, there is a lower incidence of physical and mental abnormalities, spontaneous abortions and neonatal deaths when mothers have relatively high weight gain (though not becoming obese) and babies are born heavier. It has also been shown that prolonged labors are directly related to the way in which the uterus has grown during pregnancy, and that in turn depends on how well nourished the mother has been.

During pregnancy, you should take in a broad spectrum of nutrients through a balanced diet.

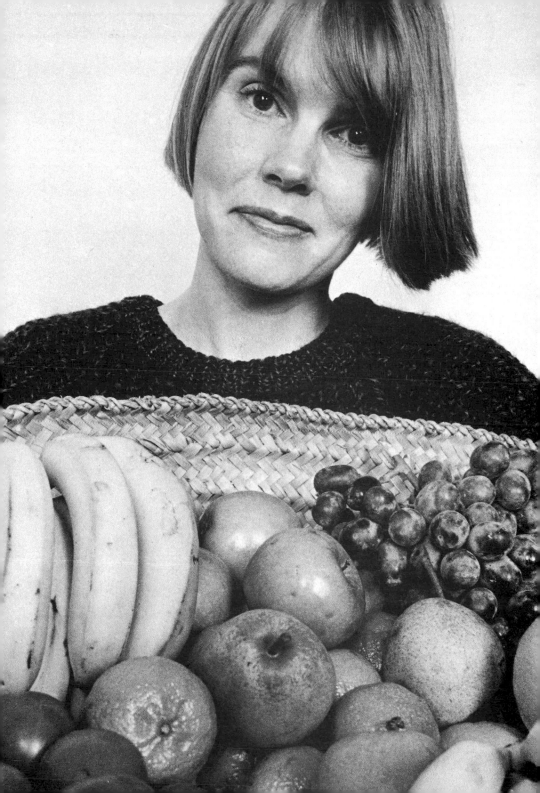

What you gain

Nowadays average weight gain is considered to be 25lb. When a woman eats what she needs, her weight gain usually follows a natural and predictable pattern. You may find you put on weight and your figure changes almost from the time you confirm the pregnancy (6–8 weeks). However, your weight gain will be monitored from around week 12 or starting with your first prenatal visit. This is the point to take note of in your calculations.

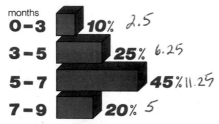

months
0–3   10% 2.5
3–5   25% 6.25
5–7   45% 11.25
7–9   20% 5

Percentage of total weight gain
This is a rough guide to your weight gain at a given time during pregnancy.

Being overweight

Although there is no ideal weight gain to aim for, that doesn't mean that you can eat whatever you want and put on as much weight as you like. Becoming obese presents several problems. For example, there is an association between excessive weight gain and Cesarean section. It's thought that when fat accumulates between the muscle fibres of the uterus they work less efficiently and cannot contract enough to finish pushing the baby out once labor has started. Obesity also puts a strain on the heart, which is already working at full stretch.

If you are definitely overweight and are on a slimming diet, it is important to stop dieting before trying to conceive. Once you are trying to conceive or are pregnant, unless your doctor considers you dangerously obese, choose the foods you eat with care but don't try to lose weight with a slimming program until you have finished breastfeeding your baby.

AWARENESS OF WEIGHT GAIN

If you run to plumpness during pregnancy, fat has a tendency to accumulate in places such as the thighs and upper arms. It is extremely difficult to take this fat off again after the birth. As this is demoralizing, here are a few tips to help you keep your weight gain within reasonable limits.

● As soon as you know that you are pregnant, get someone to take a snapshot of you, and take one every month or so after that. This reminder of your changing shape will help you keep your size in perspective. If you feel you might be putting on too much, it may help you to be strongwilled in combating cravings.

● If you've always had weight problems, but managed to keep them under control, it's easy to relapse into overeating once you know you're pregnant. Start eating sensibly from the beginning, and don't overeat in the first trimester when your appetite will increase anyway.

● Keep a supply of nutritious snacks – cheese, dried fruit and nuts, wholemeal rolls – in the house and at your place of work at all times. Avoid the high-calorie, low-nutrition foods that are so accessible, such as cakes, potato chips and soda.

● Don't eat as a way of cheering yourself up. If thinking about your baby and the birth makes you too distracted to concentrate on any serious project that would normally occupy you, try to use this extra time to develop hobbies, such as reading or embroidery. The point is to absorb your attention and break up your routine.

● When preparing meals or snacks, follow these simple rules:
– eat unprocessed foods
– include lots of roughage in your diet
– avoid fried foods
– sweeten with natural sweeteners
– cut out fattening foods.

Guidelines for eating

Most of the daily food guides for pregnant women, with long lists of items to be prepared and measured out, don't take into account how busy most women are, or that they may not always be at home for meals. Rather than worry about exact portions, or lists, you should understand *why* you need certain foods and nutrients and work out your own plan for healthy eating. If you suffer from nausea, you may also have to plan when to prepare meals.

What to eat

Your appetite will increase early in pregnancy; by the fourth month you may feel hungry all the time. This is nature's way of making sure that you take enough food for yourself and the baby. This does not mean that you can "eat for two". It's perfectly normal to eat more as your metabolism speeds up, but your energy requirements increase only about 15 per cent – 500 extra calories a day.

Every bit of food you take in should be good for you and the baby. If you ate well before you become pregnant, you should be healthy enough to get through any period of nausea (see p. 138). As your pregnancy progresses try eating a greater number of smaller meals, say five or six, instead of three more substantial ones. Small, frequent meals are always more easily digested. Bowel contractions slow down during pregnancy so the stomach empties more slowly and should not be overloaded at any one time. Your developing baby pushes up into your stomach during the last trimester, constricting its capacity, so a small meal is more easily accommodated and will leave you feeling more comfortable. The problem then arises of what sort of foods to eat as snacks. Traditional snacks such as potato chips and cookies are usually low in goodness and high in calories so be inventive, try sandwiches, nuts, fruits and soups.

FOODS TO AVOID

As a general rule foods have a higher nutritional value the less they are processed and cooked, so choosing fresh, raw wholefoods wherever you can should be your aim. Being aware of what is in food naturally, what has been added, and what has been done to it will save you from eating foods of low value or that are actually harmful. When planning what to eat remember:

● In processed foods the nutrients are either reduced, removed or destroyed by canning, pasteurizing or commercial freezing methods.

● Foods with added preservatives, flavorings and colorings contain high levels of chemicals that are undesirable for you.

● White flour products or anything containing added sugars provide little nutrition at the price of a lot of calories.

● Soft drinks contain "empty" calories and harmful additives.

● Strong coffee and tea adversely affect the digestive system; tannic acid in tea drunk with a meal can render the iron in the food unabsorbable. Caffeine and tannic acid in large quantities may not be good for the baby.

● If you consume too many manufactured, high-salt foods, such as potato chips, bottled sauces or packet soups, you may have difficulty gauging your sodium intake (see p. 103).

● Foods, such as vegetables, that are not really fresh have a reduced nutritional value.

● Certain molds produce toxic substances which you are better to avoid so watch for fruit and vegetables with diseased skins, any food that is obviously moldy, or dried foods that are stale. It is not enough to remove the moldy parts, as the harmful substances can penetrate deeper and will not be destroyed by cooking.

VITAL NUTRIENTS NEEDED IN PREGNANCY

You shouldn't need to eat much more food than you did before, but you will have to be aware of the nutrients present in the foods you choose to eat.

Protein

Your protein requirements increase by about 50 per cent, so you'll need to increase the high-protein foods in your diet. In one day this amount of protein could be gained from three eggs, 1 pint milk, ¼lb cheese, or a good helping of fish or lean meat. These foods all contain the necessary amino acids (the chemical substances which make up protein). Vegetable proteins contain only some of the amino acids so they need to be combined with animal protein or some wheat products (wholemeal bread or wholemeal pastry) to make them complete protein (see below). These vegetable proteins are found in peas, beans and lentils, brewer's yeast, seeds and nuts.

Calories

You will need about 500 more calories a day than the usual requirement of 2000–2500. Your extra calorie needs will be greater if you're having a baby within a short time of a previous one, you are still working, busy looking after a large family, underweight or under stress. You shouldn't have to concentrate on eating calories – they will come with the other foods in your varied diet.

Fiber

As pregnancy progresses there is a tendency to develop constipation (see p. 136). You can help to overcome this by giving your intestines plenty of roughage to work on. Raw fruit and vegetables, bran, whole grains, peas and beans are all fibrous foods that you should eat some of every day.

Fluids

You should not regulate your fluid intake during pregnancy, except to watch the calorie content of the drinks you take. Water is the best drink, which helps to avoid constipation and to keep your kidneys working well. If you do suffer from mild fluid retention (edema – see p. 138), you won't affect your condition by reducing your fluid intake.

VEGETARIAN DIET

Achieving a balanced diet with sufficient quantities of protein and all the vitamins and minerals requires more effort if you are a vegetarian. By eating foods in combination in order to utilize complementary plant protein sources you will gain all the necessary amino acids (see above). For example, if you are eating grains – rice or corn – combine them with dried beans or peas or nuts. If your meal is made up of fresh vegetables, add a few sesame seeds, nuts or mushrooms to supply the missing amino acids. Few people eat one food in isolation anyway.

Pregnant vegetarians who don't take any dairy products (vegans) will need to be more careful that their diet is rich in foods that contain calcium, Vitamin D (see p. 103) and riboflavin. The single problem is Vitamin B12 which is only found in animal sources. Very little is needed, but lack of it will eventually lead to a form of anemia. It can be prepared commercially from fungi and you should consult your doctor about taking this synthetic B12.

Iron is a nutrient that all vegetarians need to watch. There is relatively little of it in each helping of plant food, even leafy green vegetables and beans, and these foods often contain substances that interfere with the body's absorption of iron, so vegetarians need to eat a lot of foods that contain iron (see pp. 101–2).

Vitamins

The value of a varied and balanced diet of wholesome food is that you will take in high enough levels of vitamins without resorting to vitamin supplements. Research has shown, however, that multi-vitamin supplements, if taken before conception and during the first trimester, can prevent neural tube defects such as anencephaly and spina bifida. There are other women who doctors consider may benefit from supplements (see below).

Minerals

You are not likely to be deficient in minerals and trace elements if you eat a good diet. However, calcium and iron intakes need to be maintained and some doctors routinely prescribe dietary supplements of iron and folic acid. If supplements are not provided, ask if you need any. Your doctor may have assessed your diet and decided that it will be sufficient. It's better not to medicate yourself with supplements without your doctor knowing. So always discuss this with him or her first. Women who are nutritionally vulnerable, however, will certainly benefit from appropriate supplementation.

Calcium

A sufficient quantity of about twice your pre-pregnant intake is important from the time of conception, because your baby's teeth and bones begin to form from weeks 4–6. As your baby grows, so do your calcium requirements – by week 25 they have more than doubled. Sources of calcium include dairy foods, leafy vegetables, dried peas, beans and lentils, and nuts.

Calcium cannot be absorbed efficiently without Vitamin D. However, this vitamin is not found in great quantities in many foods; the best source is sunlight. The body can make its own Vitamin D with the help of the sun, so you don't need to worry about eating foods rich in Vitamin D (butter, milk, egg yolk, liver) unless you never expose your skin to sunlight.

Calcium supplements will be useful if you are allergic to cow's milk. You will need up to 1200mg daily in a compound form, although if you eat well 600mg should be sufficient. Vitamin D will also be prescribed and is usually given in the form of halibut oil capsules which contain Vitamin A as well.

Iron

The large increase in blood volume means that extra iron is needed to make hemoglobin for the increased number of red blood cells. The more hemoglobin the blood contains, the more oxygen it can carry to the various tissues, including the placenta. Your iron reserves will also be taken by the baby in reserve for after the birth because breast milk contains only traces of iron.

Iron is quite difficult for the body to absorb. That from animal sources (liver, egg yolk) is more easily absorbed than that in whole grains and nuts. So eating foods

NUTRITIONALLY VULNERABLE WOMEN

If any of the following apply to you, you will need to make a special effort to eat well during pregnancy. You will almost certainly need supplements as well to maintain your health and the general health of your baby, if you:
- are allergic to certain key foods, such as cow's milk or wheat
- before conception were generally run-down, underweight or eating a poor and unbalanced diet
- have had a recent miscarriage or stillbirth, or your children are spaced closely together
- drink or smoke heavily
- suffer from a chronic condition that obliges you to take some form of medication constantly
- are adolescent and still growing
- have a multiple pregnancy
- for reasons beyond your control have to work particularly hard or are subject to a lot of stress.

101

rich in Vitamin C (citrus fruit and fresh vegetables) at the same time as those that are iron-rich can double the amount of iron absorbed.

If women are iron-deficient when they become pregnant or develop iron-deficiency later on, iron tablets or injections will be prescribed to prevent the development of true anemia (see p. 61).

While it is clearly important that iron intake should be adequate, what is adequate and what form the iron should take is open to debate. The routine prescription of iron tablets (see p. 62) to a healthy pregnant woman eating a balanced diet has not been found to have any benefit for mother or baby.

Antacid medicines limit the absorption of iron, so if you suffer from indigestion and take medication, be careful about your iron intake. One good source of the mineral is iron cooking pots. Food cooked in them will absorb iron, increasing its iron content by some three to 30 times.

VITAMINS AND MINERALS REQUIRED IN PREGNANCY

Name	Food source	
Vitamin A (retinol)	whole milk, fortified margarine, butter, egg yolk, oily fish, fish liver oils, liver, kidneys, green and yellow vegetables, carrots – cooking the carrots releases Vitamin A for easy absorption	Builds up resistance to infection, essential for good vision, keeps skin and mucus membranes in good condition, necessary for the formation of tooth enamel, hair and finger nails, important for the growth and formation of the thyroid gland.
Vitamin B1 (thiamine)	whole grains, nuts, pulses, liver, hearts, kidneys, brewer's yeast, wheatgerm – don't overcook, benefits will be lost.	Aids digestion, keeps the stomach and intestine healthy, needed for fertility, growth, lactation. The body's needs increase during illness and infection.
Vitamin B2 (riboflavin)	brewer's yeast, wheatgerm, whole grains, green vegetables, milk, eggs, liver – goodness can be lost if foods are exposed to light	Helps break down all food, prevents eye and skin problems, essential at the time of conception and early days for normal growth and development of the embryo.
Niacin (B3)	brewer's yeast, whole grains, wheatgerm, liver, kidneys, green vegetables, oily fish, eggs, milk, peanuts	Builds brain cells, prevents infections and bleeding of the mother's gums.
Pantothenic Acid (B5)	liver, kidneys, heart, eggs, peanuts, wheatbran, whole grains, cheese	Essential for all normal reproductive functions of the body, maintains red blood cells.
Vitamin B6 (pyridoxine)	brewer's yeast, whole grains, liver, heart, kidneys, wheatgerm, mushrooms, potatoes, bananas, molasses, dried vegetables	Helps the body to assimilate fats and fatty acids necessary for the production of antibodies which fight disease. Deficiency causes disease of the nerves and anemia.
Vitamin B12 (cyanocobalamin)	liver, brewer's yeast, wheatgerm, whole grains, milk, soya beans, fish	Essential for the development of healthy red blood cells, necessary for the formation of the baby's central nervous system.
Folic acid (one of B complex)	raw leafy vegetables, lamb's liver, walnuts	Essential for blood formation, prevents neural tube defects, such as spina bifida, and other malformations, essential for the development of the baby's central nervous system.

Folic acid

This is essential for the supply of nucleic acids needed by the rapidly dividing cells of the embryo. As the body doesn't store folic acid and in pregnancy excretes four or five times the normal amount, enough must be taken every day. Supplements of higher doses up to 4mg are sometimes prescribed for women who have previously had babies with brain and spinal cord defects such as spina bifida. Folic acid is found in leafy vegetables and liver, but as the low doses prescribed are not thought to cause any ill-effects, folic acid supplements are worth taking for all pregnant women. Your doctor will prescribe them from about week 14.

Salt

Ordinarily most of us take in too much sodium, but during pregnancy you need more, not less salt. This need is mainly because the amount of salt in your blood is diluted by the increase in body fluids.

Name	Food source	
Vitamin C (ascorbic acid)	citrus fruits, fresh fruit, red, green and yellow vegetables – destroyed by overcooking	Helps resistance to infection, builds a strong placenta, helps the absorption of iron from the intestine, a useful detoxicant in the body, important for the repair of fractures and wound healing. Needs are variable; infection, fever and stress deplete the body's resources and cause increased needs.
Vitamin D (calciferol)	fortified milk, oily fish, liver oils, eggs, butter, egg yolk – sunshine activates a previtamin in the skin (see p. 101)	Promotes the absorption of calcium from the intestine and helps the incorporation of calcium from the blood and tissues into bone cells to strengthen the bones.
Vitamin E	wheatgerm, most other foods	Necessary for the maintenance of cell membranes, protects certain fatty acids.
Vitamin K	green leafy vegetables – manufactured by the body from bacteria in the gut	Helps in the process by which blood coagulates.
Calcium	milk, hard cheese, whole small fish, peanuts, walnuts, sunflower seeds, green vegetables	Essential for the formation of healthy bones and teeth, important in the early months when the baby's teeth are developing.
Iron	kidneys, liver, shellfish, egg yolks, red meat, molasses, apricots, haricot beans, raisins, prunes	Essential for healthy formation of red blood cells.
Zinc	wheatbran, eggs, liver, nuts, onions, shellfish, sunflower seeds, wheatgerm, whole wheat	Helps in formation of many enzymes (special proteins that oversee chemical reactions in our bodies) and of proteins, needed to ensure the release of Vitamin A from liver stores into the bloodstream.

HANDY FOODSTUFFS

A useful food is milk; though not essential it is easy to use, a cheap source of protein, and provides calcium together with Vitamins A and D. The cream in milk contains half its calories; low-fat or skimmed milk, where the cream is removed, is preferable.

If you don't like drinking milk, use it on cereals, in custards, soups and sauces, or eat cheese (two small cubes of cheddar are equal to one small glass of milk) or yogurt. If you are allergic to milk, be careful to substitute other sources of the nutrients it provides, especially calcium (see p. 101).

Potatoes are much maligned and underrated, but they are extremely nutritious, so do include them in your diet. A potato contains about 1oz of protein, together with calcium, iron, thiamine, riboflavin, and niacin, plus seven times as much Vitamin C as an apple. If you don't want to add a lot of calories, don't fry them. Try to cook them in the skins, whether you are baking, boiling whole or mashing; peeling them first means you lose a lot of fiber, most of the protein, many of the vitamins and half the iron.

You will see from the foodstuffs mentioned in this chapter that a few sources will provide the goodness you need for your own health and the growth and development of your pregnancy. Unless you are on a macrobiotic diet, your daily needs will be met by eating some of the following foodstuffs each day: milk, eggs, fish, lean meat, organ meats (kidneys, liver), yeast products, hard cheeses, wholegrain foods (brown bread, pasta or rice), fresh fruit and vegetables, fruit juices, nuts, dried fruits.

DIET AND MORNING SICKNESS

Ironically women who suffer from nausea in the first three months of pregnancy can be hungry at the same time. Food provides relief from the nausea, though the nausea soon returns. To combat this, many women find that small, frequent snacks and an avoidance of the trigger foods (usually rich, creamy or spicy foods) and smells (cigarette smoke, frying food) can help during the difficult weeks. Though called morning sickness, nausea can occur at any time of the day or even throughout the day. Work out your "good" times and prepare your meals and snacks then.

Eating more starch does seem to alleviate the sick feeling. However, this can also lead to excessive weight gain. Fat does need to be laid down in the first trimester (see p. 96), so if it's a question of eating carbohydrate in the form of a bun or cake, it's better to eat that than nothing at all, especially if you are vomiting. Try more nutritious forms of carbohydrate such as wholemeal bread, rice and potatoes, rather than pastries, cookies and cakes.

Here are some snack foods that you can prepare at home or have at your workplace to control the rising nausea during your working day.
- slices of wholemeal bread dried in the oven
- sandwiches with wholemeal bread and hard cheese
- nuts and raisins
- dried apricots
- fruit cake (preferably made with wholemeal flour and wheatgerm added)
- green crisp apples
- water crackers and cottage cheese
- raw vegetables such as carrots, celery, tender young green beans, peas from the pod, tomatoes
- fresh fruit juices, diluted with carbonated water
- carbonated water with a slice of lemon or lime
- bitter lemon or lime
- diabetic peppermints sucked slowly
- commercial muesli bars with bran, coconut or apple added
- unflavoured, natural yogurt with honey
- fruit sorbet
- herbal teas
- soft, juicy fruits such as peaches, plums and pears
- milkshakes made with skimmed milk.

DANGEROUS SUBSTANCES

As well as concentrating on what you should eat, you must try to avoid the dangerous substances that might affect your baby in the uterus.

Smoking

☐ The chemicals absorbed from cigarette smoke directly limit fetal growth by reducing the number of cells produced, in both the baby's body and brain. Nicotine makes blood vessels constrict and therefore reduces the blood supply to the placenta, interfering with the nourishment of the baby.

☐ The level of carbon monoxide is higher in a smoker's blood; whatever the woman's level, it is even more concentrated in the baby's blood. As well as being a poison, carbon monoxide reduces the amount of oxygen that blood can carry. The more carbon monoxide in the baby's blood, the lower its weight at birth. The babies of mothers who smoke can be as much as 7oz lighter than those who don't smoke, and low birthweight babies can have problems and are less likely to survive. Also the incidence of prematurity almost doubles in smokers.

☐ Smokers may eat less, so their babies may not get enough nourishment for proper growth.

☐ Studies have shown that smokers are more likely to have children with all types of congenital malformations, especially cleft palate, hare lip and central nervous system abnormalities, with the risk more than doubled in heavy smokers.

☐ Smokers have nearly twice the risk of spontaneous abortion (miscarriage and stillbirth), partly because smoking greatly increases the risk of the placenta being attached too low down in the uterus (see p. 144), and partly because smokers' placentas tend to be thinner, have damaged blood vessels and age prematurely.

☐ Neonatal deaths are more common among babies whose mothers smoked. Mothers who continue to smoke after the fourth month are increasing by nearly one third the risk of their baby dying within the first week of life.

☐ The effects of smoking in pregnancy show for a long time after your baby is born, and children who live in smoking households are less healthy. Exposure to cigarette smoke puts babies at considerable risk during the first year of life – they have a tendency to develop bronchitis and crib deaths increase.

How much?

While all smoking is thought to be harmful, the crucial level is 10 cigarettes a day, with the death rate in smokers' babies tailing off below that number. Women who cut down on cigarettes or stop smoking before week 20 tend to have

---

TIPS TO CUT DOWN SMOKING

As pregnancy causes stresses and strains anyway, you may find that you cannot stop smoking. Pregnancy can be an anxious and even boring time for some women and cigarette smoking provides the means of escape. Here are some tips to help you cut down and perhaps stop smoking altogether.

● cut down to less than 10 a day
● use the lowest tar and nicotine brand of cigarette
● always smoke filter tips
● stop inhaling
● put out a long stub – most of the tar and nicotine is in the second half of the cigarette
● if you smoke out of nervousness, occupy your hands with something else, such as worry beads
● if you need to feel something in your mouth, chew on a plastic cigarette holder (try to avoid the usual reaction of chewing on sweets or eating more)
● watch your diet – smokers may be deficient in zinc, manganese, Vitamins A, B6, B12, and C.

105

babies of a similar birthweight to non-smokers, but that still leaves the risk of congenital abnormality caused by smoking in the early stages, or even before conception (see p. 23). Women who live with smokers or are often in a smoky environment are at risk even if they never smoke themselves. Children of fathers who smoke heavily are twice as likely to have malformations.

It's particularly important that a woman who is in need of special care during pregnancy for any reason doesn't smoke because she is adding a factor that increases the possibility of something going wrong. So, if a woman has suffered a stillbirth, it is crucial that she doesn't smoke the next time she becomes pregnant as this would multiply her chances of another stillbirth.

Drinking alcohol

The extent to which alcohol, a poison, can seriously damage a developing baby has only really been appreciated in the last five or so years. Some of the alcohol out of every drink you take reaches your baby's bloodstream and is most harmful during the critical development period of weeks 6–12, although each affected growth period seems to produce its own abnormalities.

There is no safe level of alcohol consumption during pregnancy. If you are taking more than two drinks each day, there is a 1 in 10 chance that your baby will have fetal alcohol syndrome (FAS), which can lead to facial abnormalities such as cleft palate and hare lip, heart defects, abnormal limb development and lower than average intelligence. Seriously affected babies never catch up mentally or physically with their counterparts. Binge drinking can cause the same damage, even if you drink little as a rule: one incident of excessive alcohol consumption is just as capable of giving rise to FAS as drinking excessively all through pregnancy. You should, therefore, limit yourself to two glasses of spirits, wine or beer on any one day.

Some studies show that babies can be affected in less severe ways by intakes below two glasses a day. Perhaps this is because some mothers metabolize alcohol into poisonous acetaldehyde very quickly, or perhaps because some babies are genetically less resistant to the effects of alcohol – as yet no one knows. It has been demonstrated that as little as one drink a day can double the risk of having a small-for-dates baby, and babies of women drinking half that amount tend to be shorter than expected. It is beginning to be thought that very small intakes of alcohol can cause many mental conditions so far unexplained, or affect babies mentally and physically in subtle ways. Because it has not been established that any level of alcohol is *safe* for the fetus, it would seem sensible for women not to drink at all (see p. 24) once they decide to have a child, and to abstain from drinking alcohol throughout the pregnancy. Many women don't feel like drinking alcohol anyway.

Drugs

It's well known that certain drugs can affect the development of a baby, particularly at the sensitive period between weeks 6 and 12 when all the vital organs are being formed. In addition a drug may be safe in itself, but harmful to the fetus in combination with another equally innocent drug or certain foods.

Because of these dangers *no drug of any kind, and that includes aspirin, should be taken unless under the supervision of a doctor.* Don't take over-the-counter remedies for anything, or use leftover prescription drugs, or accept drugs prescribed for other people. And don't consult a doctor about anything without informing him or her that you are pregnant or trying to become pregnant.

Some drugs have to be taken for the treatment of chronic complaints (see p. 25) such as diabetes, heart disease, thyroid problems, rheumatic disorders and possibly epilepsy, but discuss the continuation of medication with your doctor before you conceive.

EFFECTS OF DRUGS ON YOUR BABY

Name of drug

Amphetamines	They are stimulants in adults and also stimulate the baby's nervous system. They may cause heart defects and blood diseases. Sometimes present in diet pills.
Anabolic steroids	All these drugs are related to male sex hormones and are used to stimulate appetite, muscle growth and weight gain. They have a masculinizing effect on a female fetus. May be present in treatments for hay fever or skin disorders. May be present in ointments prescribed for skin irritation – avoid these too during pregnancy.
Antibiotics generally	They do cross the placenta but penicillin would seem to be safe.
Tetracycline	Causes permanent yellow discoloration of the baby's teeth, may interfere with growth of bones and teeth.
Streptomycin	May cause deafness in infants. It is used to treat tuberculosis.
Antihistamines	Used to treat allergic reactions and present in some travel sickness preparations, possibly causes some malformations.
Anti-nausea drugs	Some of them have been shown to produce malformation in animal testing. It's better to try to combat nausea through your diet (see p. 104). If your nausea is very severe your doctor will know of a safe drug.
Aspirin	Can cause miscarriage if taken in large amounts. If taken in the last trimester it can affect the baby's blood-clotting mechanism and can also affect your own blood-clotting mechanism during the birth.
Birth control pills estrogen-progesterone	Can cause malformations of the limbs, defects of the vital organs and masculinization of the female fetus. Better to stop taking the pill at least three months before conceiving (see p. 26).
Codeine	Used in pain relief and in some cough medicines. Increased incidence of malformations such as cleft palate and hare lip have been reported. Is an addictive drug, can cause withdrawl symptoms in the baby at birth.
Diuretics	These are used to get rid of excess fluid from the body. They make your kidneys work harder. They can cause some blood disorders in the fetus.
Narcotics	Causes fetal addiction. Newborn babies suffer agonies of withdrawl and may need a blood transfusion after birth.
Progestogens	Some doctors may offer you tablets containing these hormones for the purpose of pregnancy testing. They cause masculinization of the female fetus so refuse them.
Psychedelic drugs – LSD, mescaline and cannabis	May cause chromosomal damage and therefore risk of miscarriage or malformations. So little is known about the effects of these drugs; try to relax with breathing and relaxation techniques (see p. 131).
Sex hormones	Sometimes given in an effort to stop miscarriage with debatable effectiveness. Can cause masculinization of the female fetus.
Sulphonamides	Can disturb the developing baby's liver function and cause jaundice at birth. Are used to treat urinary infections.
Tranquilizers	Some of the stronger types may affect growth and development, causing malformations. You could change to a milder tranquilizer but try to do without for the duration of your pregnancy.
Tylenol	A common ingredient of cold, headache and painkilling remedies. Can cause damage to the fetus' kidneys and liver. Use with caution during pregnancy.

9 Exercise

Both before and during pregnancy exercise is essential. Before you become pregnant it ensures that your body is fit to carry a healthy baby to term. Once you are pregnant it builds up strong muscles to protect your joints and spine, which slacken as a natural prelude to labor, then ache when over-used. When combined with breathing and relaxation techniques, specific exercises help you conserve your energy during labor, while others prepare you for the positions of delivery itself.

BEING AWARE OF YOUR BODY

Your body changes in many ways during pregnancy. There are the obvious physical changes (see pp. 80–89), as well as general loosening up and stretching of ligaments around the joints. But perhaps more important, from a day-to-day point of view, is the difference in what your body can do with ease in comparison to what it could do before.

In later pregnancy you become a rather ungainly shape, and because of your size you lose quite a lot of agility and mobility; you can no longer move as fast as you could without getting breathless. Your centre of gravity is further forward than usual and you find yourself less stable. Once committed to a certain direction you may find it difficult to take avoiding action, and if someone bumps into you, you may even fall over. To compensate for this lack of stability, you might hold your shoulders back, stand with your feet apart, and walk with a waddling gait.

All of these compensatory actions mean that the muscles are used in a different way from before, and you may therefore suffer minor aches and pains as pregnancy progresses. If, however, you keep your body fit during pregnancy, and are aware of how to protect it from stresses and strains, the muscles, joints and ligaments

will be able to take the strain of pregnancy more easily, without aching. You may even avoid minor discomforts altogether. Get used to thinking that your body is in a special state (not abnormal, just special), and develop reflexes and postures that take account of its needs. If you feel uncomfortable, ease your discomfort by using relaxation techniques (see p. 131).

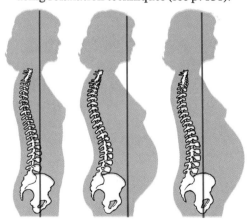

Correcting bad posture
Your center of gravity (left) is affected by the growing baby in pregnancy. There is a tendency to lean back to compensate for the increased weight (center). Good posture (right) corrects your balance and helps to avoid aches and pains.

Bending and lifting

The hormones of pregnancy soften the ligaments of the lower back and pelvis so heavy lifting should be avoided. You must protect your spine at this time and avoid unnecessary strain on your lower back when bending or lifting.

☐ Make use of your thigh muscles when lifting. Squat down first, keeping your back straight. Prepare your body (keep your feet slightly apart) by tensing the abdominal muscles, pulling up your pelvic floor muscles (see p. 112), taking a deep breath and counting to three before lifting on four. As you lift, breathe out. Stand close to whatever you are lifting and keep it close to your body as you pick it up.

☐ When you are carrying anything, avoid swivelling to either side and try to distribute the weight evenly, as for instance with heavy shopping baskets.

☐ When you are carrying your toddler keep your body straight, don't twist, and change him from side to side.

☐ If you have to do anything that involves being low down, squat (see p. 119) or get down on all fours. This is a comfortable position, particularly if you suffer from backache as it takes the weight of the uterus off your spine.

If you have bad posture, or your back isn't flexible, practice improving your suppleness by sitting cross-legged against a wall. Lengthen your spine, and do a pelvic tilt (see p. 118), pressing your back into the wall. This should help you to feel how to hold yourself well and to lengthen your spine.

☐ Avoid lifting anything heavy down from a height. Your back will arch and you could lose your balance if the object is heavier than you supposed.

PROTECTING YOUR SPINE
In later pregnancy you will need to adapt even basic everyday movements like getting up from lying down or getting out of a chair. You want to put the least strain possible on your back and let your thighs do the work.

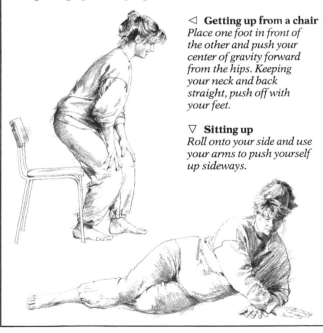

◁ **Getting up from a chair**
Place one foot in front of the other and push your center of gravity forward from the hips. Keeping your neck and back straight, push off with your feet.

▽ **Sitting up**
Roll onto your side and use your arms to push yourself up sideways.

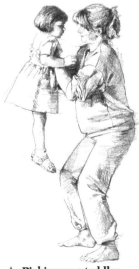

△ **Picking up a toddler**
Remember to keep your back straight and to bend your knees.

KEEPING ACTIVE

Pregnancy, labor and delivery will make great demands on your body, so the more you can prepare yourself physically, the better. Whether you do this by continuing to exercise in the way you did before pregnancy (see p. 120) or whether you embark on a new form of exercise is up to you. The important thing is to keep yourself active. The fitter you are, the less likelihood there will be of your stiffening up as pregnancy progresses. If you make sure that you sit, stand and walk in the correct ways (see p. 109), you should avoid the aches and pains that invariably come with bad posture.

The benefits of being fit

If you exercise regularly you will also find that your mental as well as your physical well-being will be helped. Exercise causes the body to release tranquilizing chemicals that help you to relax, soothing away tensions and anxiety. And the fast circulation of the blood that occurs when you exercise means that your body and your baby are well oxygenated.

Labor will almost certainly be easier and more comfortable if you have good muscle tone, and many of the exercises taught in prenatal classes, combined with relaxation and breathing techniques, will help give you more control over what is happening to you.

Keeping in condition during pregnancy will also mean that you regain your normal shape within a shorter time after delivery. Regular exercise of the pelvic floor muscles (see p. 113) will not only assist in delivery, but will also allow the muscles to regain their normal strength more quickly.

However, before you start on any exercise program in early pregnancy, check with your doctor to make sure it is safe. Some doctors feel that if a woman has a history of miscarriage or there are any complications she should not undertake exercises in the first three months of pregnancy.

When you have the "all-clear", here are a few tips for keeping fit:

□ Try to enroll in an exercise class specially designed for pregnant women. Many women find it easier to exercise regularly when they have the discipline of a teacher putting them through the exercises. It also helps to have someone watching you, correcting the way in which the exercises are done.

□ If you haven't been an active person before pregnancy you're unlikely to change dramatically during it, but at least try to walk whenever you can; 20 minutes a day is a reasonable goal.

□ Even if you have to sit down all day, there are exercises that you can do in a chair (see p. 117).

□ Get into the habit of going through a 10–15 minute exercise program every day. During pregnancy your exercises should be regular, and rhythmic whenever they can be. It's a good idea to use music when you exercise.

□ Be sure to take your exercises at a slow pace. Always warm-up gently before you start your exercise program (see p. 116).

□ Try not to go for periods with no exercise at all. Even a little exercise several times a day is better than a big burst followed by a long gap.

□ Never exercise to the point of fatigue.

□ Never do an exercise that causes you pain. Pain is a signal that something is wrong. Try a simpler variation of the exercise. Work towards a position gradually, don't strain.

□ Try not to point your toes for too long as this may cause cramps in the legs.

□ Most exercises are done on the floor and you might like to have a few pillows or cushions as aids to help you be comfortable.

□ Before each exercise, try a few deep breaths. This is relaxing, it makes you feel alert, it gets the blood flowing around your body and gives all your muscles a good supply of oxygen.

□ Swimming is easy, good exercise.

PRENATAL EXERCISE CLASSES

A variety of prenatal exercise classes is available; it is worth doing some research into what they have to offer and what type of teaching you'd be happiest with. You may be able to find the appropriate class at your hospital. Health clubs, YMCAs, YWCAs, and a number of independent organizations also offer classes.

What they teach

Some classes are run just like an ordinary exercise class, giving a thorough physical workout with exercises specifically designed for pregnant women to increase flexibility, strength and stamina. Others are designed with a certain philosophy of birth in mind. If you want to give birth in a squatting position, as Michel Odent encourages (see p. 50), there will be exercises to strengthen the back and thighs, for example. The classes are also good places for making contact with other pregnant women.

Yoga

With its emphasis on muscular control of the body, breathing, relaxation and tranquility of mind, yoga is an excellent method to use as a preparation for pregnancy. However, yoga is a philosophy which pervades the whole of life and, though special exercises for pregnancy exist, they are only a small part of the system. I think it would be wrong to expect yoga to help you in pregnancy if you are not already a devotee or have not made the effort to become one prior to your pregnancy.

Yoga exercises are comparable with some of those taught in prenatal classes but the types of breathing used are different. It is believed that these breathing techniques help to raise the pain threshold.

Being with other pregnant women gives you an incentive to exercise and keep in good condition.

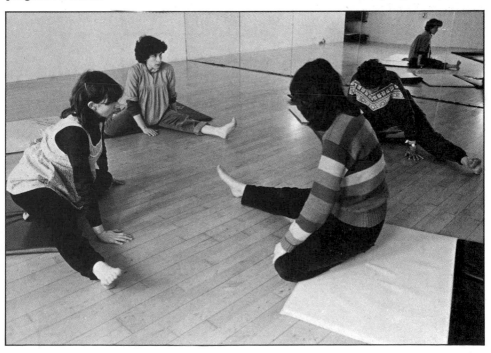

THE PELVIC FLOOR MUSCLES

These are muscles that support the uterus, the bowel and the bladder, as well as guarding the entrances to the urethra, vagina and anus. The pregnancy hormone progesterone prepares the body for birth by softening joints and ligaments and that includes the pelvic floor muscles. If pressure from the enlarging uterus causes the pelvic floor to become weak, this can lead to vague aches and fatigue, urinary incontinence and leakage, and possibly even prolapse of the uterus. About half the women who've had children suffer from some weakness of the pelvic floor, and experience discomfort or incontinence when they laugh, cough, sneeze, or lift.

To counter this, a set of exercises has been developed by physiotherapists working in the area of childbirth. They are called the Kegel exercises, after Dr Arnold Kegel of the University of California in Los Angeles, one of the first physicians to recognize how important the muscles are.

Pelvic floor exercises are recommended for all women and should begin before pregnancy and continue afterwards (they are probably even more important in older women). If you possibly can, make the exercises part of your daily routine. When exercising, do about five contractions of five seconds each. Once you've mastered the exercises, you can do them wherever you are – sitting, standing or walking – but do remember to practice as often as you can. They will also be useful in the second stage of labor when the baby's head is about to be born (see opposite).

Locating the pelvic floor muscles

Lie down with a pillow under your head and one under your knees. Cross one leg over the other and squeeze your legs tightly together. Tighten the buttock muscles and pull up as if you feel the need to empty your bladder but must wait. This helps you to locate the pelvic floor muscles, which you will feel tighten inside your vagina. Another way to locate them is to interrupt the flow of urine. When doing the exercises opposite, ignore the abdominal and buttock muscles and use only those of the pelvic floor.

Isolating the sphincter muscles

Lie down as above but with your legs relaxed and not crossed. Place a clean fingertip on the opening of your vagina and contract your pelvic floor muscles. You will be able to feel the contraction of the vaginal sphincter. The sphincter at the opening of the urethra is more difficult to isolate because of its proximity to the vagina. But it is also tightened when you contract the pelvic floor muscles.

Now place your finger at the opening of your bowels and, with a larger movement, contract the muscle around the anus. You will feel the anal sphincter tightening.

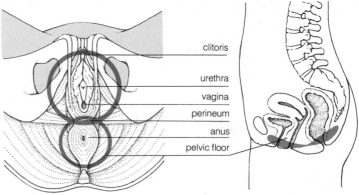

The pelvic floor muscles
These are rather like a sling that holds the pelvic organs in place (far right). They lie in two main groups forming a figure eight around the urethra, vagina and anus (near right). The layers of muscle overlap and therefore are at their thickest at the perineum.

clitoris

urethra

vagina

perineum

anus

pelvic floor

STRENGTHENING THE PELVIC FLOOR

Here are four basic Kegel exercises that will help you to strengthen your pelvic floor muscles.

Contract and release

Lie on your back with your legs apart. Draw up the pelvic floor muscles, concentrating on the muscles of the vaginal sphincter. Hold for two to three seconds then completely relax. Try to slacken a little more and notice the release in tension. Do three of these contractions in succession.

The elevator

Imagine the pelvic floor is an elevator, stopping at various levels in the store. Aim to contract the muscles gradually in five stages with a short stop at each, not letting go between levels. Then allow the pelvic floor to descend, releasing the contraction level by level. When you reach the starting point, ground level, allow the muscles to relax completely so that you feel a slight bulging downwards. If you actually push downwards, as if sending the elevator into the basement, you can lower the pelvic floor even further, and the vaginal lips will open slightly. You will have to hold your breath or blow out to feel this. This is the position in which your pelvic floor should be whenever you have an internal examination and while your baby's head is being born.

During sex

Grip your partner's penis with your vagina. Hold for a few seconds before releasing. Repeat a couple of times. Your partner will be able to tell you how hard you are squeezing and will know when the strength of squeeze is diminishing. If he says he can't feel much, then you will know that you must keep exercising.

While urinating

Start the flow of urine then stop it by pulling the vaginal muscles upwards and inwards. Hold for a count of five then let the urine flow again. Concentrate on feeling the difference between consciously controlling the flow and letting it pass automatically.

PREPARING FOR THE BIRTH OF THE BABY'S HEAD

An increased awareness of the pelvic floor muscles and how they feel when relaxed will help prepare you for the birth of your baby's head.

Exercise one

Lie on a bed with your knees bent, feet together and back supported. Press your knees together hard and tighten the pelvic floor muscles. Note the feeling of tension along the inner thighs and between your legs; many women involuntarily tense these muscles when their baby's head is stretching the outlet of the birth canal, and in fact you should try to avoid this because you are more likely to tear. Relax, and notice carefully the different feel of the muscles; this open feeling is what you should aim for when giving birth.

Exercise two

Lie on a bed, back supported with pillows but with your feet and knees apart. Gradually relax your thighs and pelvic floor muscles so that your knees fall wider and wider apart (your feet will roll gently on to their outer edges). At first this may seem unnatural and uncomfortable, but after a little practice you will get the correct feeling of letting go fully. Practice panting in this position as you will be asked to do by the midwife when it is time for your baby's head to pass slowly and gently out of the birth canal.

113

WARM-UP EXERCISES

Always precede your exercise program with some warm-up exercises. These stimulate the circulation, loosening the muscles and joints so that they move more freely, thus reducing the risk of damage. Repeat each exercise five to ten times; make sure you are comfortable and that your posture is good.

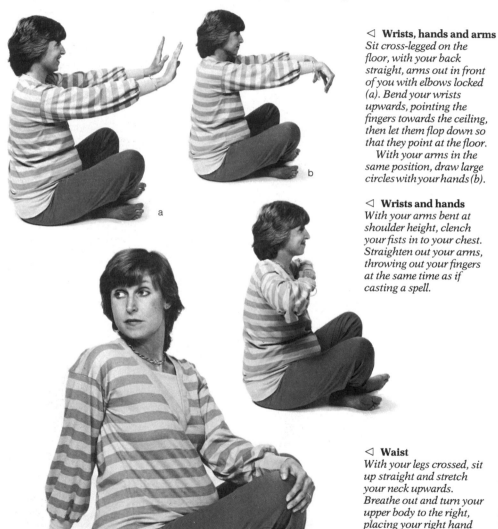

a

b

◁ **Wrists, hands and arms**
Sit cross-legged on the floor, with your back straight, arms out in front of you with elbows locked (a). Bend your wrists upwards, pointing the fingers towards the ceiling, then let them flop down so that they point at the floor.

With your arms in the same position, draw large circles with your hands (b).

◁ **Wrists and hands**
With your arms bent at shoulder height, clench your fists in to your chest. Straighten out your arms, throwing out your fingers at the same time as if casting a spell.

◁ **Waist**
With your legs crossed, sit up straight and stretch your neck upwards. Breathe out and turn your upper body to the right, placing your right hand behind you. Place your left hand on your right knee and use this hand as a lever to twist your body a little further, stretching the muscles of your waist.

Chest ▷
Sit cross-legged on the floor. Pull your hands up behind you so that the backs of your hands rest side by side against your back, aligned with the shoulder blades. Turn the palms of your hands towards each other, moving the elbows out and back. Stretch your neck up, breathing steadily, and hold for up to 20 seconds.

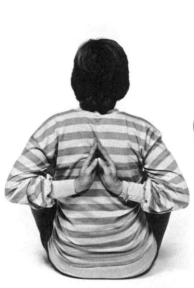

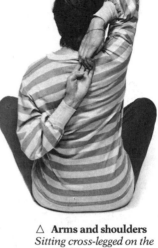

△ **Arms and shoulders**
Sitting cross-legged on the floor, lift your right arm up and stretch it to the ceiling. Bend it at the elbow and drop your hand down your back. Put your left hand on your right elbow, pushing it further down your back. Put your left arm behind your back and reach up to grasp the right hand. Stretch. Relax. Repeat with your other arm.

Legs and feet ▷
Sit up straight with your legs out in front of you, supporting your weight on your hands. Bend and straighten your knees alternately.

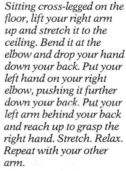

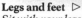

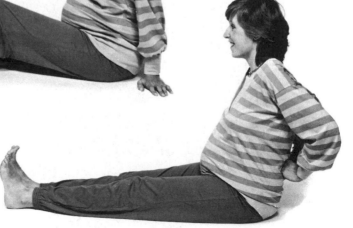

Legs and feet ▷
Sit with your legs out straight. As you breathe out, pull the toes towards your body and push your heels away, lifting them slightly. Breathe in and point the toes away. Make your hands into fists and place them in the lower back. Rub hard as you continue to point your feet up and down.

GENERAL EXERCISES

These exercises are specially designed to be useful during pregnancy and can easily be fitted into your daily life. By working on a firm surface and carrying out all the movements smoothly, you shouldn't feel any discomfort or strain. *Always* stop before you become fatigued. When you first start, repeat each exercise five times, increasing slowly by one repeat a day or every other day, until you are doing 10 or 15. The exercises can be done in any order you wish.

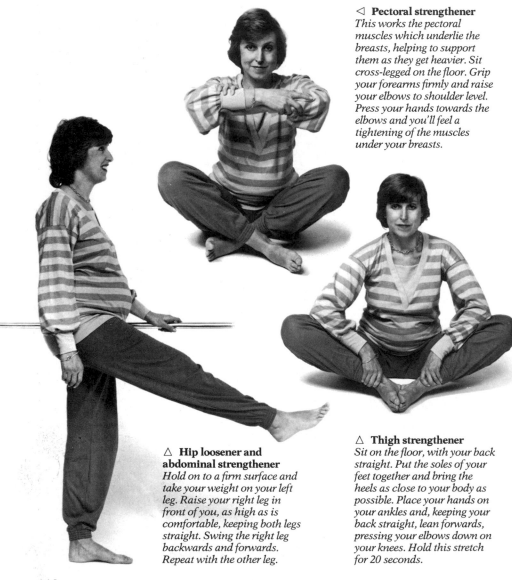

◁ **Pectoral strengthener**
This works the pectoral muscles which underlie the breasts, helping to support them as they get heavier. Sit cross-legged on the floor. Grip your forearms firmly and raise your elbows to shoulder level. Press your hands towards the elbows and you'll feel a tightening of the muscles under your breasts.

△ **Hip loosener and abdominal strengthener**
Hold on to a firm surface and take your weight on your left leg. Raise your right leg in front of you, as high as is comfortable, keeping both legs straight. Swing the right leg backwards and forwards. Repeat with the other leg.

△ **Thigh strengthener**
Sit on the floor, with your back straight. Put the soles of your feet together and bring the heels as close to your body as possible. Place your hands on your ankles and, keeping your back straight, lean forwards, pressing your elbows down on your knees. Hold this stretch for 20 seconds.

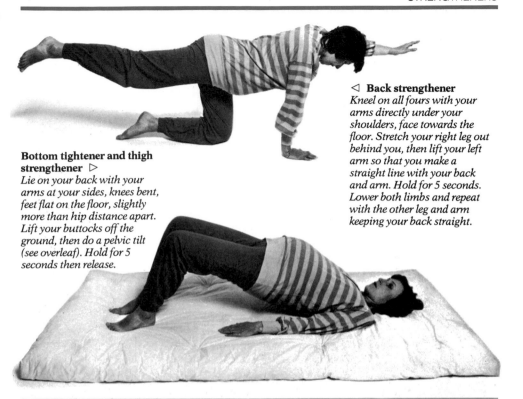

◁ Back strengthener
Kneel on all fours with your arms directly under your shoulders, face towards the floor. Stretch your right leg out behind you, then lift your left arm so that you make a straight line with your back and arm. Hold for 5 seconds. Lower both limbs and repeat with the other leg and arm keeping your back straight.

Bottom tightener and thigh strengthener ▷
Lie on your back with your arms at your sides, knees bent, feet flat on the floor, slightly more than hip distance apart. Lift your buttocks off the ground, then do a pelvic tilt (see overleaf). Hold for 5 seconds then release.

EXERCISES SITTING DOWN

While it's ideal to set aside times to go through specific routines, you can fit in a few exercises during your working day too. Try some of these stretch exercises to improve circulation. They can be done in the office or on the bus.

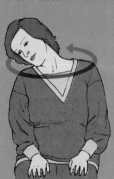

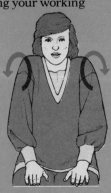

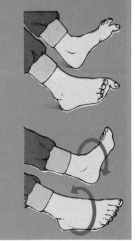

Ankle strengthener ▷
Place your heels slightly apart on the floor and bring your big toes together to touch. Turn your feet out, keeping the little toes up and the big toes down.

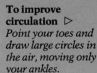

△ Head and neck
Draw circles to release tension and relax your shoulders.

△ Shoulders
Make backward circles to improve posture.

To improve circulation ▷
Point your toes and draw large circles in the air, moving only your ankles.

PELVIC EXERCISES

If you learn to move your pelvis easily during pregnancy, you will be better able to find the most comfortable position during labor. By tilting the pelvis, you strengthen the abdominal muscles, increase flexibility in your lower back and take the weight of the uterus onto your buttocks and abdomen. The pelvic tilt involves gently thrusting the pubic bone up and forwards. You can practice it standing, lying or sitting. Breathe out as you tighten the muscles and in as you relax.

Pelvic tilt lying down ▷
Lie on the floor with your knees bent and feet flat. Place one hand under the hollow of your back and the other on your hip bone. Press your back into the floor (you'll use your stomach muscles). Feel your hip bone move back and your buttocks tilt up slightly. Hold for 4–5 seconds, then release slowly. Repeat 5–10 times.

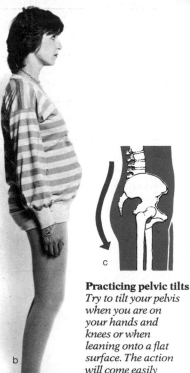

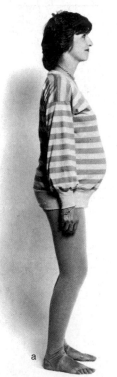

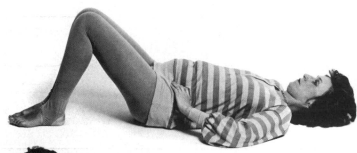

c

Practicing pelvic tilts
Try to tilt your pelvis when you are on your hands and knees or when leaning onto a flat surface. The action will come easily with practice.

◁ **Pelvic tilt standing**
Stand straight with your arms by your side. (Stand against a wall to begin with; this will help you to get the movement right.) Bend your legs slightly (a) and do a pelvic tilt, breathing out as you do (b). Your buttocks should drop down (c) as your lower back curves under. Your shoulders should remain still; only the pelvis should move. Hold for 5 seconds. Relax and breathe in. Rock your pelvis by going in and out of this position – keeping your shoulders still throughout.

a   b

SQUATTING

There are many benefits to be derived from doing squatting exercises. Squatting cuts off some blood from the general circulation and so gives the heart a rest. It makes your joints, especially the pelvic ones, more flexible, stretches and strengthens the thighs and back muscles and relieves back pain. Squatting is a comfortable position to relax in and is a practical position for labor and delivery (see p. 171). It may seem difficult at first but with practice it will become progressively easier.

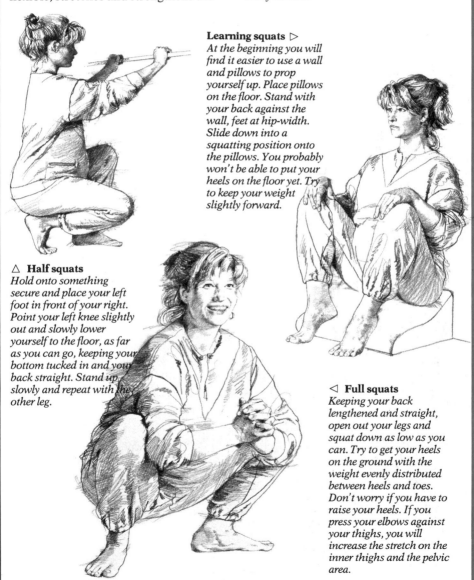

Learning squats ▷
At the beginning you will find it easier to use a wall and pillows to prop yourself up. Place pillows on the floor. Stand with your back against the wall, feet at hip-width. Slide down into a squatting position onto the pillows. You probably won't be able to put your heels on the floor yet. Try to keep your weight slightly forward.

△ **Half squats**
Hold onto something secure and place your left foot in front of your right. Point your left knee slightly out and slowly lower yourself to the floor, as far as you can go, keeping your bottom tucked in and your back straight. Stand up slowly and repeat with the other leg.

◁ **Full squats**
Keeping your back lengthened and straight, open out your legs and squat down as low as you can. Try to get your heels on the ground with the weight evenly distributed between heels and toes. Don't worry if you have to raise your heels. If you press your elbows against your thighs, you will increase the stretch on the inner thighs and the pelvic area.

SPORTS ACTIVITIES

There are several sports that you can continue to indulge in as long as you take everything at a gentle speed and stop as soon as you feel tired. Remember, if you are out of breath, your baby is also being deprived of oxygen.

Walking

This provides good exercise, so walk as much as you like. The main concern is that you walk under safe conditions.

Swimming

This provides an excellent form of exercise, and it's the one sport you can continue until term. I swam two weeks before delivery with my second pregnancy, slowly and gently of course. However, don't swim if the water is cold; you are more prone to cramp at this time.

Cycling

This will do you no harm, but you should discontinue it when your abdomen gets large enough to affect your center of gravity. You can then lose your balance more easily.

Riding and skiing

These are forbidden – even the most experienced riders and skiers can fall.

Dancing

As long as you're not too energetic and don't do acrobatics, you can dance throughout pregnancy. It's a good way to practice pelvic tilts (see p. 118).

Push off from the side of the pool and float freely on your back, arms behind your head. Try to make a star shape with your arms and legs.

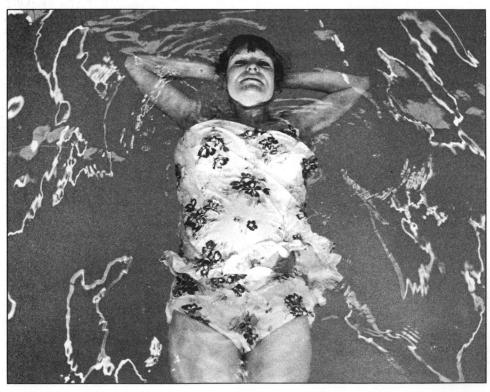

WATER EXERCISES

Swimming is wonderful exercise during pregnancy. With these exercises, you can improve your general fitness, while becoming more supple with the support of the water to help you. If you don't swim, you can still do them.

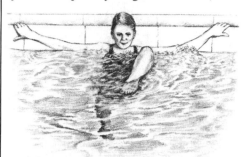

Cycling movements
With your back to the rail, hold onto it with your arms stretched out straight. Raise your legs and make slow, exaggerated cycling movements with your legs in the water. Keep cycling for a couple of minutes but don't become fatigued.

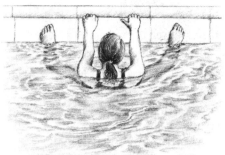

Body movements
Facing the rail, put your feet flat against the side of the pool with your knees bent. Move your body from side to side. Stretch your legs out until they are straight out to either side, feet still flat against the side, and repeat the swaying movement.

TRAVELLING

Whether you are going short or long distances, travelling is unlikely to do you any harm during pregnancy. But do use your common sense. Don't risk getting tired by taking long, unbroken journeys, particularly on your own. Resist rough and jolting cross-country trips. Don't take any travel sickness medication. Towards the end, try to stay close to home so that you are within easy reach of your doctor.

Driving

You can continue driving until your size makes it difficult to look back over your shoulder, or if the wheel jams into your stomach. For many women this occurs around the seventh month; for others there are no problems. It is illegal to stop wearing your seat belt just because you are pregnant. Some women lose their ability to make quick co-ordinated responses and to concentrate without a break during pregnancy. If you notice this happening to you, it is most unwise to drive for any distance. If you suffer from backache, make sure you have a proper support. Get out of the car at least every 100 miles and walk around in order to rest your joints and keep the blood circulation going.

Trains

Going by train is probably the most relaxing way to travel in pregnancy because there is always a bathroom close by if frequency is a problem.

Flying

At any time during pregnancy you will find travelling through time zones a strain. You shouldn't fly after 28 weeks, but if you really have to, ask your doctor, who may allow you to do so up to week 36. Eat little and often. You will be less likely to suffer from motion sickness. When travelling, always fasten your seat belt below your abdomen. During a long flight, be sure to get up and walk around frequently.

10 Looking good

In pregnancy, most women find that their skin improves as more blood flows under the skin, giving them the legendary glow and making them feel well and attractive. Pregnancy hormones have a natural, tranquilizing effect; with them you can achieve the serenity that often makes a pregnant woman especially beautiful. Exercise and a healthy diet, coupled with an awareness of the physical changes that occur in pregnancy, will contribute to your feeling happy with your changing shape. Taking care of your clothes, make-up and personal hygiene can also do a lot towards giving you a good self-image.

If you feel good, then you will probably look good too. Minimize the stresses and strains on your body by wearing comfortable, low-heeled shoes and pay attention to posture. You don't have to wear shapeless clothes; adapt your existing wardrobe for the first two trimesters.

WHAT TO WEAR

The increase in the circulation of blood throughout your body will cause you to sweat more; your vaginal secretions will also increase (see p. 142). It is therefore advisable to bathe daily (but never to douche) and to wear, whenever possible, lightweight natural fibers which won't irritate your skin or cause you to feel hot and restricted. Even in cold weather you will be astonished at how warm you feel, so wear fewer and lighter clothes than usual for your own comfort.

Keep your clothes loose fitting and simple and avoid any garments that have a tight waistband or belt or fit closely around the thighs or crotch. Most women find that up to the fifth or sixth month they can wear their regular clothes, sometimes with a safety pin or a piece of velcro to help the waistbands meet. Any garments with a drawstring or an elasticated waist can be adapted as your abdomen swells. Dark clothes will disguise your shape and a pronounced shoulder line or large neck

bows also take attention away from your stomach. Fuller clothes, such as dresses gathered at the bust or jumpers, can be worn right through to the birth; if you have enough of these you may not need to buy any special garments at all. Your breasts will also increase in size, so make sure they are not constrained in a tight bodice.

It's a wonderful boost to your morale to invest in one or two really smart or glamorous outfits, which don't need to be chosen from maternity clothes. So that you have several months to enjoy them, don't wait until your pregnancy is too advanced before going out shopping. Remember that you don't have to buy maternity clothes. From the ready-to-wear racks you should be able to find fashionable clothes to wear.

Your pregnant shape is something to be proud of and to show off; don't hide yourself away and worry about it.

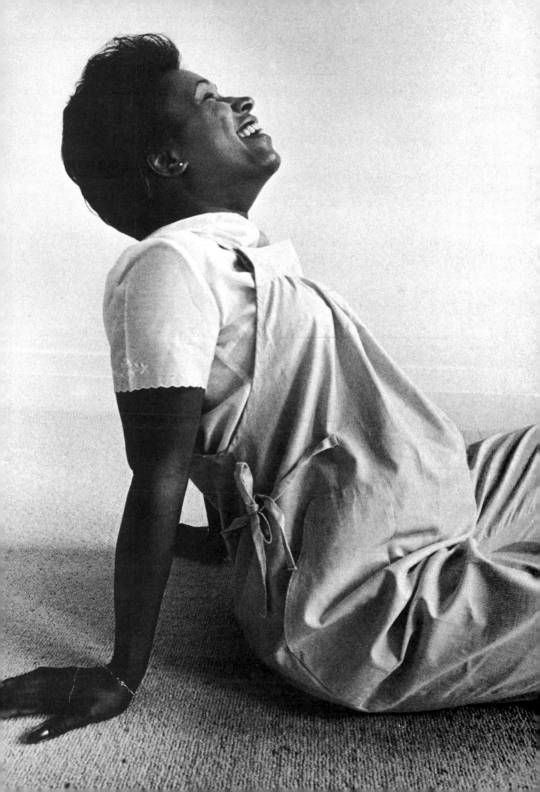

GATHERING YOUR WARDROBE

● Look in the racks of maternity clothes for ideas first and make a note of the allowances they have for expansion, such as elastic inserts and velcro strips. You can use these techniques to adapt your existing wardrobe.

● Front hems on maternity dresses tend to be 1in longer, so if you make your own or buy a non-maternity smock, check that you have the extra fabric in the hem.

● See if there is anything in your partner's wardrobe that you might borrow.

● Replace elastic in a waistband with a drawstring.

● Loose-fitting jackets, A-line coats and cloaks are the best cover-ups. A cycling cape is ideal for rainwear.

● Dresses with dropped waists are attractive.

● Don't buy too many pairs of pants; these are often uncomfortable in late pregnancy.

● Big prints and wide stripes tend to make you look larger, whereas small, flowery patterns are more subtle.

● Stretch fabrics are comfortable, but avoid clingy materials.

● On the beach an enormous T-shirt knotted on one hip or a huge scarf make attractive cover-ups.

● A layered skirt with an elastic or drawstring waistline can be worn under the armpits as a sundress, then pulled down and worn with a smock top to make a versatile summer outfit.

Footwear

Whenever you can, go barefoot. Cotton or wool socks are often the most comfortable footwear, but panty hose are fine provided that they are large and stretchy enough, do not have a tight waistband, and the feet leave enough room for your toes to move freely. If you can tolerate wearing the waistband under your abdomen, ordinary panty hose will be comfortable, but during the third trimester you may need special maternity ones. Don't wear garters, stockings, or knee-high socks with elastic tops because these tend to make the blood stagnate in your legs.

Your feet and back are going to take quite a strain as

Adaptable clothes for pregnancy

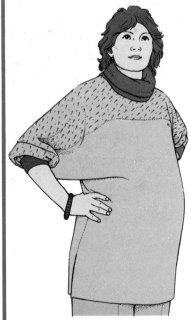

Generous sweatshirt top over loose, drawstring pants.

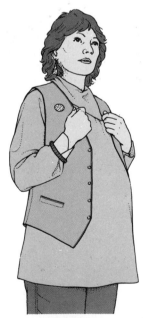

A man's vest gives a flattering layered look.

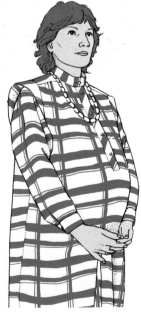

Full, elegant and comfortable smock dress.

you get heavier; your ligaments will soften and stretch. So, for the sake of foot comfort and posture, take care when choosing shoes. It is best to avoid high heels altogether, as it is difficult to stand and walk well in them. In addition they can make you unstable.

Most of the time, at least, wear low-heeled shoes that are soft and comfortable. If your feet swell, tight shoes may cut into your feet; on the other hand loose-fitting shoes can cause you to slip. Therefore, for casual wear, sneakers are excellent, though the laces may be difficult to tie later in pregnancy. For summer, canvas shoes allow your feet to swell freely.

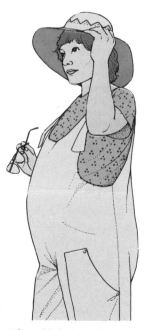

Adjustable lightweight dungarees.

Bras

You may not usually wear a bra, but you'd be unwise to avoid wearing one during pregnancy when your breasts become progressively larger and heavier, putting a strain on the supporting, non-elastic tissues. If you don't lift some of the weight from these ligaments they will stretch and your breasts will sag permanently.

From the time your breasts start to get bigger around weeks 6–8, you should wear a good, supportive bra with a deep enough band under the cups, wide, comfortable straps and an adjustable fastening. If necessary, change it for an even bigger size as your breasts enlarge. If your breasts get very heavy, you may want to wear a lightweight bra at night.

Measuring up for a nursing bra

Take the measurement directly under your breasts for the chest size and around the fullest part for the cup size.

Types of nursing bra

Both the bras illustrated below give good support, even when you are feeding.

If you are planning to breastfeed, by about week 36 you should investigate a style of front-opening bra which will allow you to feed your baby easily. Babycare shops and department stores have a wide range of styles and sizes, but if you are an unusual shape or have a narrow or wide back, see an experienced corsetier or contact one of the childbirth organizations (see p. 229). You will be wearing this bra night and day for at least six weeks. (Buy at least two.) It needs to feel comfortable, like a second skin. If you support your breasts from early pregnancy onwards, you'll probably be able to go bra-less after you stop breastfeeding, if you want to. You can buy some breast pads now in readiness for lactation.

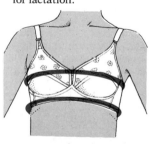

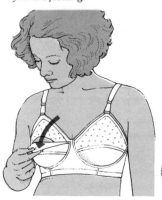

flap-opening bra

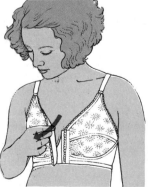

front-opening bra

SKIN AND HAIR CARE

There are good reasons for the bloom that is said to appear on a woman's skin during pregnancy. The high level of hormones in your blood (see p. 82) has a direct effect on your skin, plumping it out, helping it to retain moisture, and giving your face a smooth, velvety appearance. Added to this, your skin acquires a rosy glow because there's more blood circulating around your body. Most women's skins improve noticeably – a dry skin becoming more supple, an oily one less shiny, and any tendency to blemishes disappears. The opposite, however, can happen, and you may have to adapt your whole beauty routine. Your face may become plumper, which tends to smooth out lines and wrinkles, making you look younger and healthier or, conversely, even chubbier.

You may find that your skin itches more in pregnancy, particularly over your distended stomach. Rub any kind of oil into the skin. The oil itself may not make the difference, but the massage will certainly stimulate your blood vessels and ease the irritation.

If you have put on a lot of weight, especially on your thighs, your skin may chafe. Bathe frequently, dust the area with cornstarch or talcum powder, and keep it dry and cool. Wear cotton and avoid nylon panty hose. Calamine lotion is also soothing but the only real prevention is to cut down on your weight gain.

GENERAL SKIN CARE
- Use soap as infrequently as possible on your face and body.
- Keep hand cream and lipsalve with you to use whenever necessary.
- If you wear make-up, don't stop now; make-up is good for your skin. It slows down the water loss from the skin, helping to rehydrate it.
- Use a bath oil in your bath water. It will leave a film of lubricating oil on your skin, helping to prevent damaging water loss.

Chloasma

Any areas of skin that are already pigmented, such as birthmarks, moles and freckles, can darken, especially in olive-skinned brunettes. Sunlight will intensify this so keep covered up or use a sun block.

Occasionally brown patches (chloasma or the mask of pregnancy) appear on the face and neck. They are caused by the pregnancy hormones (see p. 82) and are often noticed in women who take the contraceptive pill. Dermatologists think that this change could be aggravated by a reaction to perfume, either as such, or in cosmetics, so test what you use. Don't try to bleach these marks out: simply cover them with a blemish stick, stippled on with your fingertips then blended and topped with a thin layer of foundation. They will go within three months of delivery. Chloasma can be brought on by sunlight and it will get worse if exposed to the sun. If you can't avoid going out in the sun, use a strong sun block. Black women may develop patches of white skin on their face and neck. These too disappear after delivery.

Spider veins

These are broken blood vessels which resemble little red spiders. They appear on the face, particularly on the cheeks. They occur when a blood vessel dilates and tiny vessels grow from this central area. They are most noticeable in fair women but disappear within two months of delivery.

Hair treatment

Some women notice a difference in their hair during pregnancy; others do not (see p. 89). It is a good idea, particularly at this time, to have your hair regularly cut in a style that is easy to care for; this will be one less thing to worry about once the baby has arrived. Wash your hair as often as you like, but if you notice a change in your hair, use the correct shampoo for your new hair condition. Take care when washing your hair that you don't damage your back by leaning over a low sink.

MAKE-UP CAMOUFLAGE TRICKS

If you wear make-up, a low-key, natural look is always flattering and makes the most of a fresh complexion. A style with startling details and bright colors won't do this. Pick a foundation tone a shade paler than the skin on your neck and a translucent powder. Stay away from pink blusher shades; shades in the apricot range are more natural. With your eye make-up, avoid hard colors – they will compete with the sparkle in your eyes – choose soft colors instead. A natural shade of lipstick will complete the effect. There are always ways to camouflage any bad points, or at least to minimize their effects.

Wrinkles

If your skin becomes drier than usual, fine lines, wrinkles and crowsfeet will look more obvious. Heavy foundations and powders accentuate this, as does anything with a shine or glitter, so abandon make-up altogether for a few days until you re-moisturize the skin, or choose the finest texture foundation you can get and a fine translucent powder.

High color

Increased blood supply can give you a permanent flushed look. To reduce this slightly, start by using a matt beige foundation with no hint of pink in it, containing quite a lot of pigment, but neither thick nor greasy in texture. With your fingertips, stipple some onto the area of the cheeks where it's needed. When dry apply a thin layer of your usual foundation on top and finish with a colorless powder. The same method is good for any tiny veins in the cheeks that become prominent, or for spider veins (see opposite). Some products sold for high-colored complexions contain green pigments. I've used these on my own rather highly colored cheeks and never really liked the results – a pasty, ghostly look.

Extra greasy skin

Use a water-based moisturizer and oil-free foundation, with translucent powder for greasy patches.

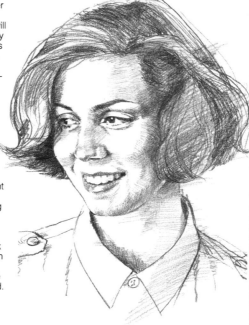

Extra dry skin

Use an oil-based film of foundation and powder. To deal with dry patches, put on two types of moisturizer; first a thin lotion that's absorbed by the skin within seconds, and on top a thicker kind that acts as a barrier to water loss. Covering with a fine layer of suitable make-up also slows down water loss. However, if your face is flaking you won't be able to camouflage it, so abandon all make-up until you have moisturized your skin really well over the course of several days. If the flakiness is accompanied by redness, see your doctor, as your skin may need special treatment.

Puffiness

This is most noticeable under the chin but can be camouflaged by shading a little brown blusher or shader subtly beneath the jawbone and on either side of the neck. To draw attention away from your jawline, try using a blusher at the temples, so that your eyes become the focus.

Dark circles

Apply a thin layer of foundation. When dry, using a thinly textured under-eye cover-up cream which you've warmed and thinned by rubbing between your thumb and forefinger, stipple over the dark areas. Leave for a couple of minutes to set, then cover with another thin layer of foundation, blending carefully. Dust with colorless powder.

Acne

If you normally suffer from pimples or blackheads, you may find that they disappear. The fluctuation of hormones may, conversely, cause you to develop acne on the face or back for the first time. This is different from ordinary acne and should not be treated with the usual proprietary preparations. Talk to your doctor if you are worried – it will usually have vanished by the second trimester and certainly by delivery.

To mask unsightly acne, stipple a little extra foundation over the area with your fingertips. If this doesn't seem enough, use the same technique to apply several thin layers of blemish stick or cover-up cream which matches your make-up exactly. Finish off with a layer of foundation, then dust with colorless powder.

Never squeeze a pimple, this will only spread germs into the deeper layers of the skin and you may end up with a hard red lump instead.

11 Rest and relaxation

During the firt three months of pregnancy you are likely to feel surprisingly tired because, although your baby is still small, your body is having to cope with dramatic changes in hormone levels. By the second trimester, however, your body will have adjusted and it is quite common to feel full of energy rather than tired. It's in the last trimester, particularly the six weeks before your baby is born, that you once again feel quite exhausted and find that you need an additional two to four hours rest out of every 24. If it is difficult or impossible to arrange a routine break during the day, just take whatever chances you get to rest or relax. If possible, do this lying down, even if you don't go to sleep. And, any time you are sitting down put your feet up if you can. If you ever feel extremely tired, don't try to fight it – give in.

SLEEP

During pregnancy it is essential to get an adequate amount of sleep; you should always aim for at least eight hours a night. Paradoxically, though, however tired and even exhausted you feel at times, you may find you suffer from insomnia. When I was pregnant with my first baby, I well remember sitting out the early hours of dawn wondering why my fatigue didn't let me sleep. I didn't know the reason for my wakefulness then, but theories now suggest that a mother's wakefulness is due to the ever-present metabolism of her baby.

A baby is growing and developing all the time, around the clock, so its metabolism doesn't slow down when evening comes – its engine keeps running at top speed. This means that the mother's body has to constantly fuel her baby with food and oxygen, and her metabolism isn't allowed to slow down. This is often reflected in her inability to sleep.

Don't fight sleeplessness and become resentful – it will only make your insomnia worse; and don't take any sleeping pills without consulting your doctor. If you can't get to sleep or keep waking up again, are restless lying in bed try some of the following tips:

□ Take the traditional remedy of a hot, milky drink.

□ Try having a fairly hot bath before going to bed. It relaxes your muscles and for many women this acts like a knockout.

□ Most pregnant women seem to need to spread themselves out when they sleep. If your bed is small it might be a good idea to invest in a larger one fairly early in pregnancy. A larger bed will also make it easier to achieve a comfortable position, propped up with several pillows, when you come to breastfeed.

□ Rather than lying flat on your back, sleep on one side in a position that you find comfortable. Get hold of some extra pillows or soft cushions and experiment with using them to make yourself more at ease. For example, when lying on your side, you might want one pillow under your stomach and another between your knees and thighs (see p. 134).

☐ Even if you have difficulty getting straight off to sleep, start going to bed earlier – you can read or do some relaxation exercises. Practice your deep breathing and concentrate on the new life inside you. Don't think of yourself as being lazy, just make sure that you get as many hours rest as you need.

☐ If you wake in the night, get up and do something that you've been persistently putting off, or do some other useful task that could save you time next day.

☐ Listen to some music, either on headphones in bed, or in another room.

If you can't sleep, don't fight it. Take a hot drink or read a book. The important thing is to rest your body and your mind.

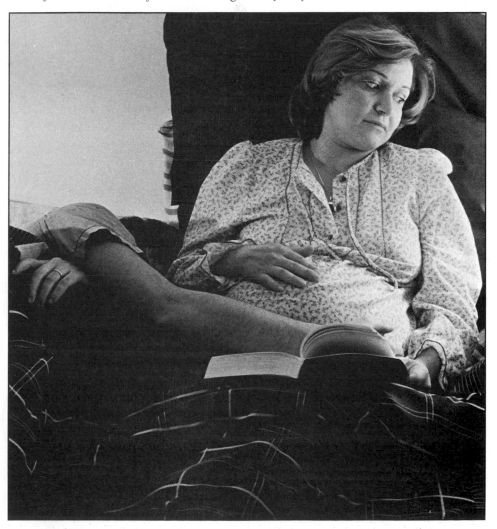

LEARNING HOW TO RELAX

Impatience, irritability, an inability to concentrate and a loss of interest in sex are all signs of fatigue. Adequate rest can cure all of them. As you cannot always expect to get sufficient sleep at night, you need to be alert to the possibilities of napping, or simply relaxing with your feet up, whenever the opportunity presents itself during the day. Long naps are not essential: five or ten minutes with your eyes closed and your feet up can be sufficiently refreshing.

Something you'll never regret is learning a relaxation technique, which, once you're accustomed to using, can recharge your batteries in a few minutes. If you want to control your body so that you can relax within 30 seconds, you might like to practice this method of instant relaxation or imagery training.

1 Arrange yourself comfortably.
2 Take in a deep breath and hold for five seconds, then count to five slowly and then breathe out.
3 Tell all your muscles to relax.
4 Repeat this sequence two or three times until you're relaxed.
5 Imagine the most pleasant thought you can. A pleasant scene is a good one (see opposite). This helps you to use your imagination and to break down your mental blocks so that you can get more in touch with your body. Learning to control your body will be useful during labor and childbirth.

Rest whenever you can; don't wait until your body aches all over and tiredness compels you to lie down. You can rest with your toddler in the middle of the day while he has a quiet play.

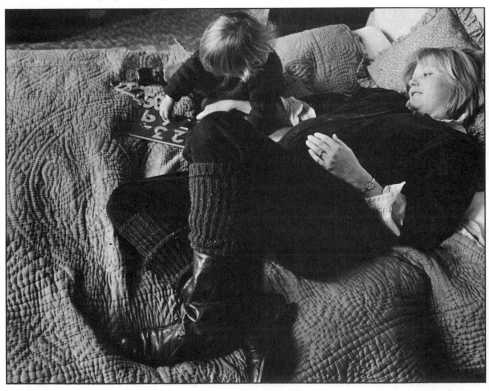

RELAXATION TECHNIQUES

Physical relaxation

This method involves giving orders in sequence to release the tension in different parts of your body. This is best learnt through tensing and then letting go. You will feel the difference in labor when you should be able to relax most of the muscles in your body and let the uterus contract without the rest of your body tensing. Your partner can help you by touching you where he can see you are tensing up; you can respond to his touch by letting go.

It is best to practice this drill twice a day for 15–20 minutes if you can. Practice just before meals or an hour or more after eating.

1 Find a comfortable position lying on your back or propped up with cushions.
2 Close your eyes.
3 Think about your right hand; tense it for a moment, let it go, palm upward.
4 Tell your hand to feel heavy and warm, press your elbow into the floor or cushions, let it go.
5 Now work up through the right side of your body, through the forearm, the upper arm, into the shoulder. Raise your shoulder, let it go.
6 Repeat on the upper left side of your body. Your hands, arms and shoulders will feel heavy and warm.
7 Roll your knees outwards, relaxing your hips and press your lower back gently into the floor or cushions. Release and let the relaxation flow into your abdomen and your chest. Tell the muscles to feel heavy and warm.
8 Your breathing should start to slow down. If it doesn't, slow it down by counting to two between each breath.
9 Now relax your neck and jaw. With your lips together, drop your jaw with your tongue on the bottom of your mouth with your cheeks loose.
10 Pay special attention to the muscles around your eyes and in your forehead, smoothing away any frowns.

Mental relaxation

Once you have mastered the technique of muscle relaxation you can try relaxing your mind in this way.
1 Try clearing your mind of any stressful thoughts, anxiety or worry by breathing in and out slowly and regularly. Concentrate all your attention on your breathing actions, even saying to yourself very slowly "breathe in, hold, breathe out."
2 Let pleasant thoughts flow through your head and freely associate.
3 If any worrying thought recurs, prevent it from doing so by saying "no" under your breath or return to concentrating on your deep breathing.
4 With your eyes closed, imagine a tranquil scene such as a clear, blue sky or calm, blue sea. Try to visualize something pleasant and blue because this has been found to be a particularly relaxing color.
5 Think fairly hard about your breathing and become aware of it. Feel how it is slow and natural. Concentrate on each breath as you inhale and exhale. Listen to your breathing.
6 You should be feeling calm and restful by now – it might be helpful to repeat a soothing word or mantra such as love, peace or calm, or you may prefer a word with less symbolism such as breath, earth or laugh. Think of a word or even a calming sound like "aah" while you are breathing out.
7 Remind yourself to keep the muscles of your face, eyes and forehead relaxed and tell your forehead to feel cool.

It might help you to settle into your relaxation method if you adopt a starting routine. For example, if you repeat a mantra or drop your shoulders this can be the signal to the rest of your body to begin. Whenever you practice a relaxation method, make sure that you are breathing deeply, in the most controlled way (see overleaf).

BREATHING TECHNIQUES

A large part of your time in prenatal classes will be spent learning how to relax and master the different breathing techniques. It's important to learn different levels of breathing; you will be able to use each one at different times during labor to help you to relax, conserve energy, control your body and pain and to calm you and prevent you from being fearful. Once you realize that you can exert a high degree of control over your body just through concentrating on breathing, you will have confidence when you go into labor and apply the same techniques. Here are three basic levels that will help you. If you practice them with a friend or your partner, you can identify the correct level more precisely.

Deep breathing

When you breathe in you should feel the lowermost part of your lungs fill with air and your lower ribcage expand outwards and upwards. If someone places their hands on your lower back when you are sitting comfortably, you should be able to move their hands with your inhalation. It feels like the end of a sigh and is followed by a slow, deep exhalation. This produces a calming influence and is ideal for the beginning and end of contractions.

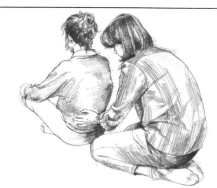

Light breathing

Aerate only the upper part of your lungs so that the top part of your chest and your shoulder blades lift and expand. Your friend can feel this if she places her hands on your shoulder blades. Your breaths should be fast and short with your lips slightly apart. Draw the breath in through your throat. After ten or so light breaths you may need to take a deep breath. This level of breathing is used at the height of a contraction.

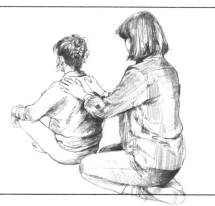

Panting

The lightest method of breathing I found most useful was panting. This is taking shallow breaths and resembles what you see and hear when a dog pants. Think of this as "pant, pant, blow." One of the times when you will be asked to pant is during transition, to stop you bearing down before the cervix is fully dilated (see p. 169). When you're taking short, rapid, shallow breaths, the diaphragm is contracting and relaxing quickly and this prevents you from making a downward, concerted push. It's also useful to pant right through a painful contraction as you won't feel out of breath at the end. To stop overbreathing, or hyperventilating, you should pant 10–15 times and then hold your breath for a count of five.

MASSAGE

Physical contact is a source of comfort and solace at any time, but more especially during pregnancy. Massage can be a means of relaxing you, bringing you and your partner close together; it's also useful in the first stages of labor to relieve back pain and to reassure, calm and soothe you.

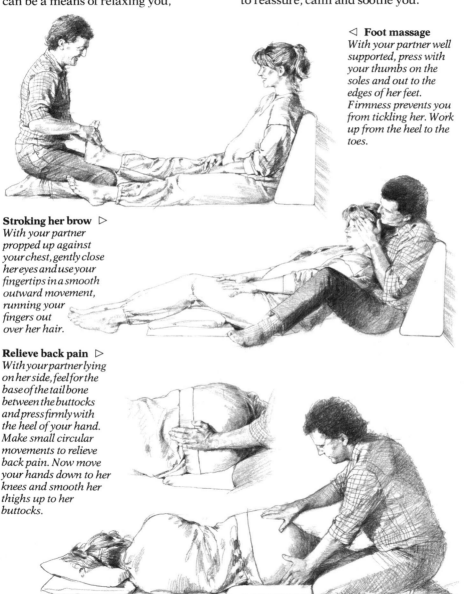

◁ **Foot massage**
With your partner well supported, press with your thumbs on the soles and out to the edges of her feet. Firmness prevents you from tickling her. Work up from the heel to the toes.

Stroking her brow ▷
With your partner propped up against your chest, gently close her eyes and use your fingertips in a smooth outward movement, running your fingers out over her hair.

Relieve back pain ▷
With your partner lying on her side, feel for the base of the tail bone between the buttocks and press firmly with the heel of your hand. Make small circular movements to relieve back pain. Now move your hands down to her knees and smooth her thighs up to her buttocks.

COMFORTABLE POSITIONS

As your abdomen gets larger, sitting or lying in your usual positions can become uncomfortable. If you lie flat on your back for any length of time, especially in later pregnancy, the weight of the baby will press down on major blood vessels running up your back. This can make you feel uncomfortable and dizzy as your

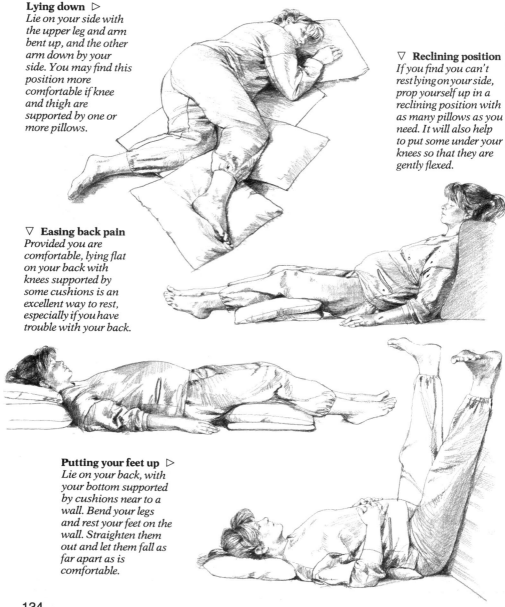

Lying down ▷
Lie on your side with the upper leg and arm bent up, and the other arm down by your side. You may find this position more comfortable if knee and thigh are supported by one or more pillows.

▽ **Reclining position**
If you find you can't rest lying on your side, prop yourself up in a reclining position with as many pillows as you need. It will also help to put some under your knees so that they are gently flexed.

▽ **Easing back pain**
Provided you are comfortable, lying flat on your back with knees supported by some cushions is an excellent way to rest, especially if you have trouble with your back.

Putting your feet up ▷
Lie on your back, with your bottom supported by cushions near to a wall. Bend your legs and rest your feet on the wall. Straighten them out and let them fall as far apart as is comfortable.

blood pressure drops; it can also aggravate hemorrhoids. It's not advisable to sleep this way but a short rest or exercising on your back shouldn't cause problems. Pillows and floor cushions help too, but don't lie with too many pillows under your head or your spine will be too curved. When sitting, don't cross your legs or have them tightly bent as this may aggravate varicose veins. Instead try some of the positions given here and be constantly aware of maintaining good posture.

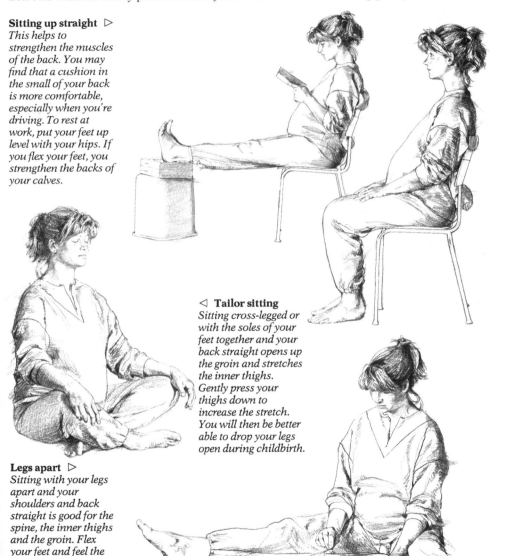

Sitting up straight ▷
This helps to strengthen the muscles of the back. You may find that a cushion in the small of your back is more comfortable, especially when you're driving. To rest at work, put your feet up level with your hips. If you flex your feet, you strengthen the backs of your calves.

◁ **Tailor sitting**
Sitting cross-legged or with the soles of your feet together and your back straight opens up the groin and stretches the inner thighs. Gently press your thighs down to increase the stretch. You will then be better able to drop your legs open during childbirth.

Legs apart ▷
Sitting with your legs apart and your shoulders and back straight is good for the spine, the inner thighs and the groin. Flex your feet and feel the stretch along your thighs. Make sure you keep your knees and toes pointing upwards.

12 Common complaints

COMPLAINT	CAUSES
Abdominal pain **2, 3**	Round ligament pain occurs during pregnancy when the ligaments supporting the uterus stretch.
Backache **1, 2, 3**	Progesterone causes softening and stretching of the ligaments, most importantly in the pelvic joints. The ligaments supporting the spine also relax, which puts extra strain on the muscles and joints of the lower spine, pelvis and hips. Bad posture can make backache worse.
Bleeding gums **1, 2, 3**	The gums thicken and soften due to the influence of the pregnancy hormones and the increased blood supply to all parts of the body. They swell, especially around the margins of the teeth. Food tends to collect in the hollows around the base of the teeth, allowing bacteria to grow and multiply and cause tooth decay and possibly gum infection (gingivitis).
Constipation **1, 2, 3**	Progesterone causes relaxation of the muscles of the intestine and thus slows down bowel movements. Bowel contents tend to stagnate and dry out so that the stools become hard and painful to pass.
Cramps **3**	Thought to be a result of low levels of calcium in the blood. In rare cases it is a lack of salt in the diet.
Cravings **1, 2, 3**	Thought to be related to high levels of progesterone.
Discomfort in bed **3**	As a result of indigestion or heartburn (see overleaf) or, when you lie down, the enlarging uterus presses on the diaphragm, stomach and ribcage.

The bold numbers following each complaint refer to the trimester (a trimester is one third of a pregnancy) in which the problems are most likely to be experienced.

While most women have normal, healthy pregnancies, there is no denying that pregnancy can be an uncomfortable time. Many of the problems are irritating rather than any real cause for concern; a lot of aches and pains can be explained away as a combination of tiredness and carrying around that extra weight.

SYMPTOMS	TREATMENT
Either stabbing cramp-like pain when you get up after sitting or lying for a time or a dragging pain on one side only.	None. Pain normally spasmodic so pain killers not worthwhile. Hot water bottle to relax muscles.
General ache across the lower back. Sacroiliac pain is classically across the top of the buttocks and extending down into them.	Good posture and exercises to strengthen the spine (see p. 117) to make it more supple. Very high heels on shoes may make it worse. Wear sensible shoes with a moderate heel. Have a good firm mattress on your bed. Avoid heavy lifting (see p. 109). If the pain runs down your leg towards the foot, consult your doctor in case of a slipped disc. Try to avoid analgesics. Massage (see p. 133) may help.
Bleeding from the gums after brushing or eating hard foods. General tenderness of the mouth. Gingivitis causes more bleeding than is normal after brushing.	Attention to oral and dental hygiene is essential, with regular brushing of the teeth after eating. Visit your dentist regularly, but tell him or her you are pregnant, as you should avoid X-rays at this time. There is no truth in the tale that the baby takes calcium from your teeth. Gingivitis should be reported at once to your dentist.
Infrequent hard stools. Pain in the lower abdomen.	Obey the call to empty your bowels whenever your body tells you. Take plenty of dietary fiber and lots of fluid, preferably water. Regular exercise helps too. Avoid strong laxatives.
Pain in the thigh, calf and foot, sufficiently painful to wake you and make you cry out. A hard knot of pain often followed for some hours by a general ache.	Very firm massage, possibly for several minutes; it also helps to flex the foot up and push into the heel. If cramp persists, see your doctor, who may prescribe calcium tablets.
Strong desire for certain foods which prevents sleep or relaxation.	Indulge yourself provided the foods aren't fattening.
Shortness of breath, acid regurgitation, soreness and tenderness of the ribs.	Try sitting up with two or three extra pillows or try some of the positions on p. 134. Get a firm bed and avoid heartburn (see overleaf).

COMPLAINT	CAUSES
Edema 3	Increase in the amount of fluid retained by your body and stagnation of this fluid in the lower parts of your body and your fingers. Pressure of the uterus on the blood vessels that return blood to the heart from the lower parts of the body.
Fainting 1, 3	Pooling of the blood in the legs and feet when standing, together with the demands of the uterus for an increased blood supply, causes the brain to be relatively deprived of blood.
Flatulence 1, 3	Unwittingly swallowing air and after eating certain foods, e.g. beans, fried foods and onions. In pregnancy the intestine is more sluggish and the gas may be more difficult to expel.
Heartburn 3	The valve at the entrance to your stomach relaxes in pregnancy, allowing small amounts of acid to get into the esophagus (the tube running from your mouth to your stomach).
Incontinence 3	Pressure of the enlarging uterus on the bladder, reducing its capacity, and the inability of the pelvic floor muscles to stop leakage when you cough or laugh.
Insomnia 1, 2, 3	The general increase in your metabolism. The baby doesn't distinguish between day and night, so it may kick you at night. Also frequency of micturition and sweating may cause you to wake.
Micturition (urination) 1, 3	Early in pregnancy the blood supply to the whole pelvis is increased causing the bladder to become irritable and to empty itself more frequently. Later in pregnancy the weight of the uterus on the bladder reduces its capacity.
Morning sickness 1	Sudden high levels of hormones, particularly the human hormone chorionic gonadotrophin (HCG), the production of which closely parallels the time of nausea. It is not clear though why it affects some women and not others. Diet before conception can predispose to nausea in early pregnancy, particularly a diet low in vitamins, minerals and carbohydrates. Tiredness also contributes to making nausea more severe, though it is not a direct cause.
Nasal discomfort 1, 2, 3	Softening and thickening of the mucus membranes in the nose. Increase in blood to the lining of the nose due to high levels of pregnancy hormones. You may wake with a blocked nose in the morning. Rough blowing may rupture tiny blood vessels.

SYMPTOMS

TREATMENT

SYMPTOMS	TREATMENT
Swelling of the hands and ankles. Shoes feel tight. Your fingers may feel stiff in the morning.	Avoid standing, particularly in hot weather. Rest with your legs up, and rest at least once during the day. Avoid very salty foods. If you have severe edema, your doctor may restrict your salt intake.
Dizziness, spinning, unsteadiness and need to sit or lie down.	Avoid standing still for long periods of time. Don't jump up from sitting too suddenly. Take care when getting out of a hot bathtub. Keep yourself as cool as possible in hot weather. If you feel faintness coming on, lie down with your head flat and if possible raise your legs slightly.
Distension of the intestine, rumbling of the stomach, frequent passing of gas.	Try not to gulp air and avoid problem foods. Hot drinks may help.
Burning sensation behind the breastbone sometimes accompanied by the regurgitation of sour fluid.	Avoid the foods that experience shows give you trouble; don't eat a meal just before going to bed. Prop yourself up in bed and try a warm milk drink. Antacid medicines (see p. 102) may be prescribed.
Leakage of urine whenever you increase pressure within the abdomen when you bend down, laugh.	Empty your bladder often and avoid heavy lifting and constipation. Do your pelvic floor exercises regularly (see p. 113).
Difficulty going to sleep, or getting back to sleep after waking.	Wear light night clothes to avoid overheating. A hot milk drink or a hot bath (see p. 128) before bed may help. Try a good book. Rarely will doctors prescribe sleeping pills except in the last trimester if the problem is leading to exhaustion.
Urgent need to pass urine, even the smallest amounts, and at frequent intervals day and night.	Nothing much you can do except reduce your liquid intake before going to bed. Later in pregnancy, try rocking backwards and forwards as you pass urine. This lessens pressure on the bladder; it may be more completely emptied. If you have any pain or blood when passing urine, see your doctor.
Feelings of nausea at the sight or smell of food, or cigarette smoke. Occasionally accompanied by vomiting.	Eat little and often and avoid those foods that make you nauseous. Don't get overtired as this will make your nausea worse. If you understand why you are feeling ill, and appreciate that it will pass, you may be more tolerant and more relaxed about it. Try the diet ideas (see p. 104), suck peppermints or nibble dried fruits, or crackers, and keep up your fluid intake. Talk to other women; if you know you're not the only one it may help. Your doctor will be loathe to prescribe anything for you.
Stuffiness in the nose, unexpected nose bleeds, congestion upon waking, snoring or runny nose.	Treat your nose gently. Avoid dry dusty atmospheres. Don't use a nasal spray without talking to your doctor. For a nose bleed, apply gentle pressure to the bridge of your nose. Lean forward slightly.

COMPLAINT	CAUSES
Pelvic discomfort 3	The baby's head presses upon nerves, causing pain in the groin, particularly when it is engaged in the pelvic cavity at the end of pregnancy.
Pigmentation 2, 3	Increased production of melanocyte stimulating hormone (see p. 82). Made worse by exposure to strong sunlight.
Piles, 2, 3	The pressure of the baby's head in the pelvis in late pregnancy may obstruct the blood vessels in the rectum, impairing the return of blood from the pelvic organs and causing ballooning of the veins around the rectum. If one of your parents had piles, there is a possibility you will get them too. Anything that increases pressure in the abdomen, such as constipation, chronic coughing or lifting, will worsen piles.
Rashes 3	Excess weight gain, poor hygiene and sweating in the folds of the skin.
Rib pain 3	Costal margin pain results from the compression of the ribs as the uterus rises, the high position of the baby's head and excessive kicking by the baby.
Shortness of breath 3	Pressure on the diaphragm prevents free excursion during inhalations and exhalations. Lying down can also push the uterus and baby up against the diaphragm.
Stretchmarks 2, 3	Depends on your skin type, and its elasticity. However, whatever your skin type, excess weight gain may cause stretchmarks (see p. 88).
Sweating 2, 3	Increased blood supply causes the blood vessels beneath the skin to dilate (see p. 86).

SYMPTOMS	TREATMENT
Pain in the groin and down the inside of the thighs, particularly bad after walking or exercising. Pins and needles spreading down the back of your legs to your feet. Also may be some discomfort where the pubic bones meet at the front.	Rest, avoid violent exercise and take an analgesic such as Tylenol but consult your doctor first.
Darkening of the skin around the nipple and areola, down the centre of the abdomen (linea nigra), deepening of any pigmentation in freckles or birth marks, mask across the face (butterfly mask) and down the sides (chloasma).	Use sun blocks when out in strong sunshine. Never bleach the skin. The pigmentation will fade within a few months of delivery.
Itching, soreness, severe pain when passing stools, slight blood loss if the pile is large and prolapses outside the rectum.	Prevent piles with a diet high in roughage, plenty of fluids and exercise, thus avoiding constipation. Keep your stools soft and regular. Try not to strain when you move your bowels. Minor piles will get better after delivery, but if they persist you may need soothing creams. Keep the anal area clean to avoid irritation. If piles itch badly, apply an ice pack or crushed ice in a plastic bag.
Intertrigo is a red skin rash occurring where heavy folds of skin become irritated by sweat. Usually found under heavy breasts or in the groin area.	Keep areas with rashes clean and apply a soothing lotion such as calamine, or try talcum powder. Keep your weight under control if that is the problem.
Soreness and tenderness, usually on the right side. Felt just below the breasts. Severe when sitting up straight.	The pain will disappear as soon as the baby's head drops into the pelvic cavity prior to birth (or earlier in some women, particularly first-time mothers). Try not to compress the ribs, prop yourself up or lie down.
Shortness of breath on exertion or just from talking.	Be less active, rest more and save your breath by not talking too much. If accompanied by chest pain, consult your doctor.
Silver marks on the skin of the thighs, abdomen and breasts.	Creams and ointments will have no effect. Eventually the marks will become smaller, narrower and a light silver color, but they rarely disappear altogether. Make sure you do not put on too much weight too quickly.
Intense perspiration on a little exertion. Waking at night in a lather of perspiration.	Wear light cotton clothing and cotton underwear. Drink more to replace lost fluids.

COMPLAINT	CAUSES
Taste 1, 2, 3	Thought to be related to the pregnancy hormones.
Thrush 1, 2, 3	The yeast Candida albicans infects the vagina. Why it is more common in pregnancy is not known. Can infect the baby's mouth at birth.
Tiredness 1, 2, 3	Sometimes because of worry, lack of sleep (see insomnia), poor nutrition, and towards the end of pregnancy the sheer burden of carrying around the unborn baby.
Urinary tract infection (cystitis) 1, 2, 3	Slackening and relaxation of the muscle wall predisposes the bladder to infection at any time during pregnancy. The high level of progesterone is again the cause. Symptoms may appear gradually over several weeks or months.
Vaginal discharge 1, 2, 3	Increased blood supply to the vagina and cervix and softening and thickening of the mucus membranes results in an increase of normal mucoid discharge. Brown or yellow discharge could be a sign of cervical erosion; the increased secretions may result in an ulcer in the vagina near the cervix. This ulcer could be damaged during sexual intercourse, and spots of blood, not of a continuous nature, may appear.
Varicose veins 1, 2, 3	A family history of varicose veins may mean that you develop them too. Near to term the baby's head can press down on the pelvic veins causing blood to pool in the veins of the legs and the result is ballooning of these veins. Standing for long periods of time will make them worse. Sitting with tightly crossed legs cuts off blood flow. Excess weight gain also causes the veins to dilate. Varicose veins on the vulva may result if the baby's head is interfering with the flow of blood there. The vulva then becomes swollen and congested.
Visual disturbances 1, 2, 3	Retention of fluid. If contact lenses feel different, this is because the eyeball has slightly changed shape with the increase in fluid.

SYMPTOMS	TREATMENT
Often a metallic taste. Appreciation of the taste of certain foods alters. Coffee, alcohol and spicy foods, for example, become less palatable than before. Often increased liking for sugar and sweetness.	None.
Thick white vaginal discharge accompanied by intense itchiness. Can be some pain when passing urine.	Antifungals in the form of a suppository and a cream will be prescribed. They clear up the infection in two to three days. If the baby contracts the infection at delivery, a course of medication will quickly clear it up. Try not to wear tight underpants.
Desire to sleep at odd times. Need for more sleep at night. Legs ache and seem unable to carry you any further later in pregnancy.	Avoid overactivity. Sleep or rest whenever you can. Eat small meals and often to keep up your energy. Go to bed early. Get others to do the work.
Increased desire to pass urine. Discomfort and pain. Urine may contain spots of blood. Dull discomfort in the lower abdomen.	Drink plenty of water. See your doctor. Your urine will be tested and you will be given specific anti-infectives to eradicate the infection.
Slight increase over normal of the clear, white discharge, which does not cause soreness, pain or irritation.	Do nothing. Don't douche or use a vaginal deodorant; don't use too much soap. Wear a light sanitary pad if it troubles you. If spots of blood appear, inform your doctor.
Skin may be irritated or itchy at first, or a dull aching pain felt. Then the veins appear as dark purplish lines on the legs. A heavy feeling in the vulva.	Avoid standing for long periods of time. Wear support panty hose, put them on before you get up in the morning after lying with your feet raised for a few minutes. Sleep with your feet on a pillow. Do exercises to improve circulation in your legs and feet (see p. 115). For varicosity of the vulva, sleep with your bottom on a pillow or wear a sanitary pad firmly against the swollen part.
Long or short sightedness may develop. Contact lenses may be uncomfortable to wear.	If you notice anything different, go to an optician. If you wear contact lenses, tell your doctor. You may have to stop wearing them during pregnancy.

13 Special-care pregnancies

Not every pregnancy is textbook but it's quite wrong to view some events, such as a multiple pregnancy for example, as abnormal. Rather they are variations of the normal which require special care. Other concerns, like diabetes, can be pre-existing medical conditions that you have to learn to cope with during your pregnancy. Yet others, like miscarriage, are true complications of pregnancy. For any unforeseen problems there may be warning signs; speedy consultation with your obstetrician may avert a tragic mishap. No one will blame you for being anxious and needing reassurance. Medical staff are unanimous in their desire to have early notification of any problems.

ANEMIA

Pre-existing anemia is no preclusion to pregnancy – more than 90 per cent of women may be slightly anemic before they become pregnant. The commonest form of anemia is due to loss of blood at menstruation which leads to iron-deficiency anemia (when the hemoglobin level is less than 12–14gm/100ml blood – see p. 61). Before you become pregnant a wise precaution would be to consult your doctor, who can correct iron-deficiency anemia very simply with a course of iron supplements. You can also increase your intake of iron-rich foods.

BLEEDING IN THE THIRD TRIMESTER

Before 28 weeks, bleeding from the vagina can be a sign of a miscarriage (see p. 148). After this time the fetus is considered viable: that is, it could survive outside its mother's womb. Any bleeding after 28 weeks is known as third trimester bleeding. The two main causes of this bleeding derive from the placenta and are known as placenta abruptio, a very rare condition in which part of the placenta comes away from the wall of the uterus; and placenta previa.

Placenta previa

This is when the placenta is located over or very near the internal os of the cervix, instead of being attached to the upper part of the uterus. There is no known cause for this rare condition, which occurs about once in 167 pregnancies. The onset of bright red blood is not accompanied by any pain.

Placenta previa may be detected early on in pregnancy by an ultrasonic scan, which will show the shadow of the placenta lying in the lower curvature of the uterus. Once this complication is confirmed, meticulous medical care is called for. If your condition is unstable, for example, if you are bleeding, you will have to remain in the hospital until delivery. If the placenta is placed extremely low in the uterus, covering the cervix, there will certainly be more bleeding before the

WARNING SIGNS
You should notify your doctor immediately if you have any of the following symptoms; while you are waiting, rest in bed. If you cannot reach your doctor for whatever reason, call an ambulance and alert the doctor's office that you are coming into the hospital.
- Very severe nausea or vomiting several times within a short period
- Vaginal bleeding
- Severe headache which doesn't go away, particularly in the second half of pregnancy
- Severe abdominal pain
- A fever of 100°F or over regardless of the cause
- A sudden reduction in the amount of urine you pass, for example if you don't urinate for 24 hours even though you're taking in normal quantities of fluid during that time
- Rupture of the membranes
- Absence of fetal movement for 24 hours from the 30th week of your pregnancy onwards
- Sudden swelling of the ankles, fingers and face
- Sudden blurring of vision

onset of labor and bleeding as soon as labor starts. In severe cases Cesarean section will be performed and this happens to about six out of every ten women with placenta previa in the United States of America.

DIABETES

Most women who are diabetic have straightforward, normal pregnancies. As it's essential for your health and that of the baby to keep your diabetes stable and under good control, you'll be seen more frequently than usual by your doctor and you'll be kept under close medical supervision. You will need to pay special attention to your diet. Your doctor will control your drug requirements carefully, as they may vary during pregnancy. With modern prenatal care, complications such as pre-eclampsia (see p. 150) are now becoming very rare.

The presence of sugar in your urine (see p. 60) doesn't necessarily mean you're diabetic. Quite often pregnancy has the effect on the kidney of letting sugar filter through from the blood to the urine; this can be normal. Special blood tests will be done to determine whether or not you do in fact have diabetes.

ECTOPIC PREGNANCY

This means that the ovum which was fertilized in the Fallopian tube fails to reach the cavity of the uterus. Instead the ovum is for some reason trapped in the Fallopian tube and grows in its cavity. An ectopic pregnancy doesn't proceed for long because the tube will eventually burst. Before it bursts there are symptoms that signal all is not well. Besides a positive pregnancy test, there is pain in the lower abdomen, usually on one side (the side of the tube in which the pregnancy is developing); there may be vaginal bleeding; and sometimes there is fainting.

If you have any of these symptoms you should call your doctor.

Surgical treatment is mandatory; the pregnancy must be removed from the Fallopian tube. Sometimes it's necessary to remove the whole tube depending on how much damage has been done. Research has shown that fertility is reduced after one ectopic pregnancy.

The incidence of ectopic pregnancy has possibly increased due to the insertion of IUDs. A coil-induced inflammation of the tube means that the egg can go no further on its journey to the uterus.

HEART DISEASE

Women with pre-existing heart disease often have easy pregnancies and labors; some women even experience an improvement in their heart condition. Nowadays heart disease is not considered a bar to pregnancy except for women who have serious limitations of normal life. You'll be closely supervised during pregnancy and you must take great care to rest so that no extra strain is put on the heart. Extra rest should include at least two naps during the day and 12 hours sleep at night. If you get a chest infection, or your temperature rises, or you notice swelling of the hands, face or feet, you should go to bed and call your doctor.

HYPERTENSION

This is another name for raised blood pressure. Blood pressure is given as two figures, for example 120/70 (see p. 61). Doctors are more concerned about a rise in the lower number, the diastolic pressure which is a measure of the heart pumping when you are at rest. As pregnancy can cause a rise in blood pressure, if you know that your blood pressure is raised, you should consult your doctor before becoming pregnant (see p. 25). There is no reason why, after all the tests are considered and with proper prenatal care, you should not have a normal pregnancy and labor, though you are more likely to be admitted to the hospital early.

Raised blood pressure in later pregnancy can be one of the early signs of pre-eclampsia (see p. 150). The difficulty with taking blood pressure readings is that anxiety and stress, perhaps caused by a long wait in the doctor's office or because you know you are prone to raised blood pressure anyway, may mean that the problem appears worse; your reading may be high as a result of your emotional state. It would be wise to rest often and curtail physical exercise so that strain on the heart is minimized. If you become anxious at the doctor's office, practice your relaxation techniques (see p. 131) to calm yourself down.

INCOMPETENT CERVIX

Under normal circumstances the cervix remains closed so that the fetus is retained in the body of the uterus and doesn't fall into the vagina. If the end of the cervical canal is open this is described as an incompetent cervix. This condition is very rare unless the cervix has been previously injured or has been damaged during surgery or pregnancy. A previous difficult or rapid labor where the baby was very large may cause it. Surgical procedures such as an unskilled abortion may also damage the muscle fibers which hold the cervical opening closed. However, the cause is unknown.

Usually an incompetent cervix remains hidden until the first miscarriage has occurred. The cervical canal starts to open by the 14th week and by the 20th has dilated to about 1in, which is large enough for the bag of waters to bulge into the cervix and eventually break. There is usually a sudden loss of water, followed by a miscarriage with little pain.

A special stitch is inserted around the cervix to tighten it; this is known as a Shirodkar or McDonald suture. This can be performed before or during the next pregnancy. The cervix is usually stitched during pregnancy, around the 14th week, under a general anesthetic. This treatment has a high success rate and most pregnancies proceed normally. At term the stitch is removed without anesthetic. Labor usually begins shortly afterwards either naturally or by induction, but some women do go a week or so longer before they have their baby.

MULTIPLE PREGNANCY

Twins are either identical – formed from a single egg – or non-identical – formed when two eggs are fertilized. Identical twins share the placenta. It may be difficult for doctors to be sure that you're carrying twins, but they will be alerted if:

● there are twins in your family

● your uterus is consistently bigger than your dates suggest

● two fetal heartbeats can be picked up with an electronic fetal stethoscope

● as pregnancy advances, two heads can be felt as well as multiple arms and legs.

Ultrasound will confirm the presence of two babies. Twins are usually diagnosed for certain by week 8 of your pregnancy.

You will have special prenatal care with an emphasis on avoiding anemia (see p. 144) through regular blood checks, assiduous checking of blood pressure to make sure it doesn't rise; and plenty of rest to keep your blood pressure low, which helps to prevent the uterus from going into labor prematurely. A multiple pregnancy puts extra pressure on your joints and ligaments and on your digestive organs. Any irritating minor symptoms such as flatulence and dyspepsia should be

TWIN PRESENTATIONS

The most common presentation for twins is for both to be in the cephalic position (left). This should present no problems at delivery. If one baby is breech and the other cephalic (right), the cephalic baby will usually be born first and will open up the birth canal so that the second baby should be delivered easily. If both babies are breech, if one baby is lying transversely, that is across the womb, or if the babies are large, a Cesarean section may be the safest course.

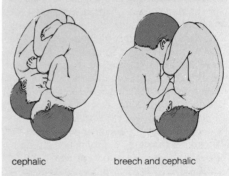

cephalic   breech and cephalic

promptly attended to. Because the uterus may crowd out your digestive organs, eat little and often. Salads and light nutritious snacks will prevent you becoming too uncomfortable. If you take care not to gain too much weight and pay particular attention to posture most complications can be avoided.

The large size of the uterus can also cause shortness of breath, piles, varicose veins and abdominal discomfort. At the first sign of any of these symptoms alert your doctor and you'll be given help, advice and treatment. You may suffer from more nausea in the first trimester, but this is by no means the rule. You will probably have to have your babies in a hospital because of the risk to the second baby if it isn't born immediately after the first baby.

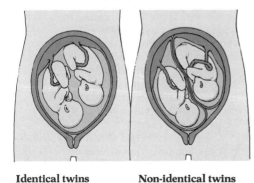

Identical twins
These develop from the fertilization of one egg that splits into separate cells. They are always the same sex and look alike. They share a placenta but have their own cords and sacs.

Non-identical twins
These are the result of two eggs being fertilized by two sperm. They each have their own placenta and need be no more alike than any two children in the same family.

147

MISCARRIAGE

Sometimes called spontaneous abortion, this is the term used when the fetus is discarded by the uterus before the 28th week of pregnancy. After the 28th week, it is called a stillbirth (see p. 200). Doctors use the words abortion and miscarriage synonymously; medically speaking, there is absolutely no difference between them, despite the fact that for many people abortion connotes that the miscarriage has been induced, whereas a miscarriage is something that occurs spontaneously. Overall the frequency of miscarriage may be as high as one in ten pregnancies, but it is first pregnancies that are more likely to miscarry – about one third of all first pregnancies abort. This is thought to be for two reasons: first, a young uterus needs to mature by having a trial run before it is ready to carry a pregnancy to full term; and second, it is thought that the majority of these miscarriages are due to a defect in the sperm or the ovum, resulting in an abnormal fetus.

The majority of miscarriages, however, occur during the first trimester. Most of these pregnancies would never have developed properly, revealing a deformity or a malfunctioning placenta. Indeed, many miscarriages occur before the woman is even aware that she has conceived and is therefore pregnant.

Miscarriages can be caused by the following conditions:
- an incompetent cervix (see p. 146)
- an incompatible blood type which develops antibodies to your partner's blood type, causing fetal death
- an hormonal deficiency so that the uterine lining is insufficiently developed to support and nourish the developing fetus
- an anatomical problem of the uterus so that it is not formed to carry a pregnancy, or uterine fibroid tumours
- placental insufficiency – if the placenta is not functioning well or has not developed properly it cannot adequately nourish the baby
- diabetes

IF A MISCARRIAGE THREATENS
- Call your doctor and go to bed.
- If you pass any clots or membranes, or the fetus and the placenta, collect them in a clean container for the doctor to examine.
- Don't take any medicines or alcohol.
- Lie flat if the bleeding seems heavy and keep your room cool.

What happens

Miscarriage is nearly always heralded by bleeding from the vagina, with or without abdominal pain. An early miscarriage may cause no more discomfort than a menstrual period without cramps. In some instances vaginal bleeding does not mean that a miscarriage will inevitably occur, but since there's no way of knowing this, consult your doctor.

As far as a doctor is concerned, any bleeding during the first 28 weeks of pregnancy is considered to be a threatened abortion until proved otherwise. The bleeding may be light or heavy, accompanied by the passage of mucus or not, and there may be a small amount of backache and discomfort in the lower part of the abdomen. Doctors have come up with no better explanation for a threatened abortion in the early stages of pregnancy than "hormone imbalance" or a "hormone insufficiency" which doesn't suppress the next period. If bleeding of this type occurs and the hormone levels remain low, miscarriage will almost certainly follow.

The treatment for a threatened abortion is some bedrest. This increases the blood supply to your uterus. When bleeding has stopped, activities should still be sensibly restricted until the 14th week of pregnancy. It's best to abstain from coitus and strenuous exercise until fetal movements have been felt at about 20 weeks with a first baby and 18 weeks with second and subsequent babies.

TYPES OF MISCARRIAGE

Threatened abortion
An abortion is possible but not inevitable; bleeding from the vagina, is rarely accompanied by pain.

Inevitable abortion
Vaginal bleeding is accompanied by pain due to the uterus contracting. If on internal examination the cervix is dilated, an abortion is bound to occur.

Complete abortion
The fetus and the placenta have been expelled from the uterus.

Incomplete abortion
The fetus has been lost but some of the products of conception are still in the uterus and must be removed surgically.

Missed abortion
The fetus is no longer alive but is still in the uterus. The fetus will be expelled by the uterus eventually.

Recurrent abortion
An abortion has occurred on more than one occasion, for different reasons and at different stages of the pregnancy.

Habitual abortion
Three or more miscarriages have occurred at the same time and possibly for the same reason in each pregnancy. High temperature and abdominal pain following abortion indicate infection.

Inevitable abortion

If the bleeding does not stop, and if abdominal pain appears or worsens, usually meaning that the uterus is contracting to expel the fetus, most medical experts agree that efforts should not be made to salvage the pregnancy.

If the miscarriage is incomplete, you will need surgical attention. Examination of the products of conception doesn't always reveal that part has been left behind in the uterus, but this becomes obvious when bleeding persists after the miscarriage has taken place. It's important to have the uterus cleaned out to avoid further hemorrhage and pelvic infection. This involves admission to the hospital for a dilation and curettage operation under a general anesthetic. The cervix is stretched and any abnormal materials are removed from the uterus.

Emotional effects

Miscarriage at any time, but particularly one in the second trimester of pregnancy, has a profound psychological effect on a woman, not just because of the loss of the baby and the mixed emotions resulting from that, but also because of the sudden withdrawal of pregnancy hormones without the reward of having a baby.

There are many fears – about your own inadequacy, that you may never be able to carry another baby, that your fertility may be permanently affected, that you had an abnormal baby this time and that you could have another next time. I also think that there is a feeling of real bereavement. I suffered a miscarriage myself at 14 weeks and was actually shown the fetus, which was well enough formed to distinguish that it was a boy. For about six weeks afterwards I found myself in a deeply depressed, depersonalized state, unwilling to communicate with other people or participate in day-to-day activities. It's normal to feel anger and grief, but you shouldn't feel guilt – it really isn't your fault, and although you may feel like being alone, try not to isolate yourself.

When to start the next pregnancy

This, of course, is a matter of choice and planning, but sexual relations can begin as soon as the bleeding has stopped. There are no medical reasons to wait, and my advice has always been to try to forget the first mishap and to start a second pregnancy as soon as you both want to.

PRE-ECLAMPTIC TOXEMIA (PET)

Rarely occurring before the 20th week, pre-eclamptic toxemia has no known cause, although it has been associated with poor nutrition. Pre-eclampsia usually develops slowly, hence the necessity for regular prenatal visits. If it is allowed to continue without intervention, the blood pressure will continue to rise, headaches will develop, there will be visual disturbance, mental dullness and in the late stages even fits. The risks to the unborn baby will increase as the blood pressure rises. There is a possibility of a premature labor because of placental insufficiency (see p. 148) and reduced chances of survival for the baby.

The best treatment is prevention, but if pre-eclampsia has developed, the treatment is admission to the hospital, bedrest, sedation and monitoring of kidney function and blood pressure. Only in rare instances does pre-eclampsia fail to get better but should it not do so, it will be necessary to perform a Cesarean section. If your blood pressure falls below 90 and remains constant, you may be allowed

SIGNS OF PRE-ECLAMPSIA
Doctors will be alerted if two of the following are present:
1 Raised blood pressure – an increase which would ordinarily be so small, but in pregnancy is considered abnormal. For example, a diastolic blood pressure of 90 would not be regarded seriously in a non-pregnant woman, but in pregnancy, it should be around 60 or 70.
2 Protein in the urine – signifies early damage to the kidneys.
3 Swelling of the feet, ankles or hands – swelling of the face may also be present; it can be part of a general weight gain but swelling due to fluid can usually be recognized as there is also puffiness around the eyes and neck.
4 Excessive weight gain.

home after four to five days. Very soon after delivery, the swelling goes down, blood pressure returns to normal and the kidneys regain their normal function.

RH BLOOD INCOMPATIBILITY

At your first prenatal visit a specimen of blood will be taken so that your blood group is ascertained (see p. 61). Besides the standard ABO blood grouping, you will be given a Rhesus blood grouping, either positive or negative. Special attention is given to Rhesus negative mothers.

Rhesus negativity is much less common than Rhesus positivity; about 80 per cent of the population are Rhesus positive. If your partner has Rhesus positive blood the chances are that you'll carry a Rhesus positive baby. As a Rhesus negative person you will perceive Rhesus positive blood as foreign; and if you're ever exposed to it, for instance by a transfusion, you will develop antibodies to Rhesus positive blood cells which will kill them. During pregnancy, blood cells from your Rhesus positive baby may escape across the placenta into

your own circulation; your body will try to destroy them with Rhesus positive antibodies. This is likely to happen at delivery. With your first baby there is little danger because you are being exposed, probably for the first time, to Rhesus positive blood cells; as a result the level of your Rhesus antibodies is low. They may even be absent unless some of your first baby's blood enters your circulation at birth and you react by forming antibodies.

Danger during subsequent pregnancies can be insignificant because antibodies may never be formed in large enough quantities. However, at various points during your prenatal care doctors will take the precaution of finding out what level of antibodies is present in your blood. It's known that a certain level of antibodies may damage the developing baby, this

The first pregnancy

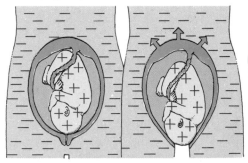

The mother's blood

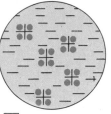

Subsequent pregnancies

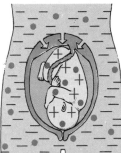

● Rhesus antibodies
— Rhesus negative
+ Rhesus positive

How RH incompatibility occurs *During the first pregnancy there is rarely a problem (above left) unless the maternal and fetal bloodstreams mix. If some of* *the baby's Rhesus positive blood cells escape into the maternal bloodstream (above), it reacts to form Rhesus antibodies (above right). In* *subsequent pregnancies, any Rhesus antibodies may cross the placenta and damage the baby's blood (above) if it is Rhesus positive.*

level, however, is reached in less than 10 per cent of women who are Rhesus negative. Don't be despondent, therefore, if the doctor tells you that you have Rhesus negative blood. In practical terms all it may mean is that you get extra special care.

Beating RH blood incompatibility

This complication of pregnancy is becoming less and less common; after the birth, a Rhesus negative mother has a blood test to see if any of the baby's cells have entered her circulation. If they have, she will be given an injection of anti-Rhesus globulin which destroys any of the baby's cells remaining in her blood so that no more antibodies can be produced. Provided this is done after every delivery or abortion, when possible leakage of fetal blood to the mother might occur, future babies are safe from RH blood incompatibility. Babies whose mothers have not had this treatment will be closely watched. All hospital obstetric units are expert in dealing with this situation. You may have one or more amniocentesis tests (see p. 68), and if by chance the baby is affected, an intrauterine transfusion may be carried out.

It may be decided that your baby should be born before term, in which case a

Cesarean section will be done. In a few cases the delivered baby may need a blood tranfusion to replace its own blood cells, which have become damaged during pregnancy. Very occasionally all the baby's blood must be exchanged, especially if jaundice is present. Paradoxically your baby will be given Rhesus negative blood though it has Rhesus positive blood itself. Some of your Rhesus antibodies may still be in your baby's body and would further damage Rhesus positive blood if it were transfused. As a Rhesus positive baby cannot produce antibodies to Rhesus negative cells, the transfused blood cells will die over a period of time and be replaced by the baby's own healthy Rhesus positive blood cells. During the transfusion about 1/3oz of your baby's blood is withdrawn at a time, and the same quantity of fresh blood is transfused back into the baby. In as little as 72 hours your baby will have gotten rid of all the antibodies that have been passed on from you; after the third day there is generally no need for any further transfusions to be carried out. Once your Rhesus antibodies and the yellow pigment which causes jaundice, bilirubin, have been "washed out" of the baby's system, it will come to no further harm and be a perfectly normal, healthy child.

14 Preparing for the birth

By the 36th week of your pregnancy, you may have given up work and should be slowing down your social and domestic routines. You may feel frustrated and bored or you may welcome the rest from your work routine or feel energized and want to spring clean the house from top to bottom. This is the time to check that everything – the room, the clothing, the equipment – is ready for the new arrival, and to prepare yourself, your partner and your other children for the birth.

ORGANIZING YOUR HOME

There are many things you can do to prepare yourself and the household to cover your day-to-day routine and to make life easier for you after the baby is born.

□ If you don't already have one, and you can afford it, buy an automatic washing machine. It will make the extra work so much easier, particularly if you choose cloth diapers. A dryer is handy too.

□ Start to neglect certain parts of your domestic life. Allow the non-essentials to slide and don't worry about them.

□ Stop doing any housework that involves hard physical effort.

□ Make sure that your family realizes that you can't dash around as you used to. Get others to help with errands.

□ Try not to worry about things that don't matter. The highest priority is the baby that is growing inside you. Try to judge your pace and don't overdo anything.

□ Sound out a reliable neighbor who will help in emergencies.

□ If you have a freezer, stock it with staple foods that freeze well such as bread, butter and vegetables.

□ Buy supplies of dried foods and the essentials such as detergent, toilet rolls and disposable diapers.

Getting the baby's room ready

If you have enough space, you can give the baby a separate room and make it into a nursery, but this isn't absolutely necessary – your baby's space can be a corner of a larger room. In the early weeks after delivery you will probably have the baby with you in your bedroom or in an adjoining room for most of the 24 hours and will use the nursery very little. After that it is ideal to have a room that is specially designed and equipped for all the baby routines such as feeding, bathing, changing, dressing and playing.

There is no need to go to a lot of expense. Your baby will grow quickly and require different things in a short time, so there is little point in investing a great deal of money in baby equipment. Before long you'll be adapting the nursery to a toddler's bedroom. Most of the equipment can be purchased second-hand. Look around in local papers and shop windows or ask your friends.

If you furnish the nursery only with the essential items, you can then add any other things when you have the practical experience of handling your baby.

Nursery equipment

● Bassinet and crib – a bassinet is a luxury for the first few months. Your baby can just as easily sleep in a Moses basket, which has other uses, or in a carry crib. A tiny baby can sleep in a crib but put up protective bumper pads of padded fabric all around.

● Moses basket – this soft wicker carrier can be useful for up to six months depending on the size and vigor of your baby. An advantage of the Moses basket is that you can carry it with you as you move about the house, thus never having to be too far from your baby.

● A firm, flat mattress with a waterproof cover–babies should never have pillows as they might suffocate in the fabric covers.

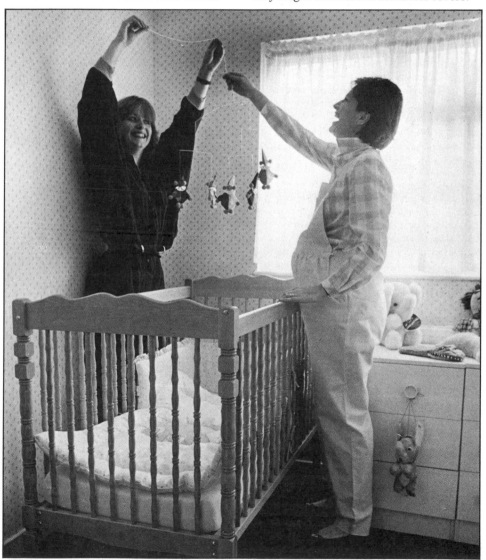

- Fitted flannel sheets for warmth – at least 4–5.
- Quilt and/or cotton thermal blankets – a tiny baby gets lost under a quilt. The blankets are better at first; even if the baby burrows down in them, she can still breathe through them.
- Muslin diapers for catching spit-ups and protecting your clothing during burping sessions. They can also be stretched across the crib under the baby's head to catch any spit-up and protect the sheet.
- Diapers – you will need to opt for either diaper buckets and laundry or disposables. Studies have shown that when cloth diapers, diaper sterilant and electricity for the washing machine are added up, disposables are not that much more expensive. You must decide. Use disposables for the first few weeks to give yourself a break from the washing. If you use cloth diapers, buy at least two dozen good-quality diapers. Cheap, thin ones will not last the necessary two years. If you choose cloth diapers, you will also need 2 plastic buckets with lids, and diaper pins – at least 4–6.
- Diaper liners – these don't have much effect on the diapers of tiny babies. Their stools are too liquid and pass through. They can be reused after washing.
- Plastic pants – these are even useful with disposable diapers as they keep in the wet. For cloth diapers you will need at least 6 pairs. They quickly become brittle and crack. So buy the best quality and try to wash out by hand, not in the machine.
- Portable bath – this isn't essential. The baby can be bathed in the kitchen sink or bathroom basin. A big bath may be rather frightening for her at first.
- Plastic changing pad.
- 2 soft new towels – your own towels will feel like sandpaper against the baby's perfect skin.
- Natural sponge or soft washcloths.
- Cotton balls.
- Vaseline, cleansing lotion, toilet rolls or baby wipes for changing time.
- Baby lotion or baby oil for flaky skin.
- Blunt-ended scissors.

- A diaper bag – this cloth and plastic bag unfolds to reveal a waterproof area for changing the baby and pockets all around that hold diapers, change of clothes, cleansing lotion and diaper pins. It can then be rolled up and slung over your shoulder after the diaper change.
- Stroller or carriage – you will have to do a lot of research here to decide on your needs. For the first few months a carriage can be a good way to give the baby "outings," but not if you have to maneuver up and down steps. If you have a car and drive everywhere, a folding "umbrella" stroller may be perfect. If you travel on

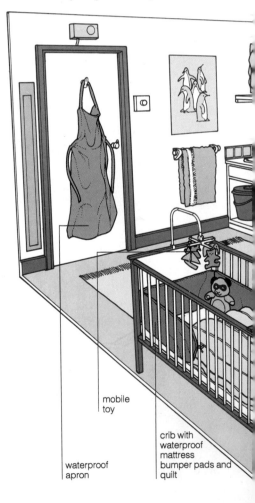

mobile toy

waterproof apron

crib with waterproof mattress bumper pads and quilt

public transport, a stroller that adjusts to the horizontal position is ideal. There are so many designs now, shop around and ask other mothers.

● Front carrier and back pack – the front carrier is for the first six months or so depending on the weight of the baby. A back pack can also be useful once the baby can sit up. He will enjoy peering over your shoulder on your outings.

● Feeding equipment if you are not breastfeeding.

● Infant seat – in this reclining seat the baby can be partly propped up and can see you moving around the room.

ESSENTIAL BABY CLOTHING
● 6 stretch suits – you may be showered with tiny clothes for the baby. The first size only lasts about 6 weeks but you will need a lot.
● 2 nightgowns – these make diaper changing easy.
● 4 undershirts with envelope necks.
● 2 cardigans or jumpers – lacy patterns are impractical as they catch around little fingers.
● 2 pairs cotton socks or booties.
● 1 shawl.
● 1 bonnet.

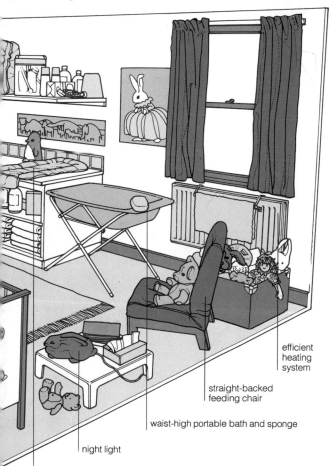

efficient heating system

straight-backed feeding chair

waist-high portable bath and sponge

night light

sink unit with changing pad, baby's toiletries, diapers

Decorating the nursery
See that all the surfaces in the nursery are hygienic and easy to wipe clean. Use only a non-toxic, lead-free paint. Make sure that there is plenty of storage space, especially around the changing area. If you are adding any units, save expense by not fitting doors. You can see everything at a glance and reach in without opening cupboards or drawers. You'll probably need doors later though when your baby becomes more mobile and inquisitive.

The floor covering ideally should be linoleum or cork tiles. A dimmer switch is a good idea for night feeds. The heat control is also important; the temperature should be constant at around 70°F. If this is too hot for the rest of the house, install a thermostatically controlled heater in the nursery.

For your comfort you'll need a low feeding chair and table. It may be a bit of a luxury, but if it's at all possible install a small sink with running water in a corner of the room.

155

PREPARING FOR LABOR AND BIRTH

The hospital or your midwife will give you a list of the items you will need for your labor and birth. If you are having your baby at home, you will need to prepare a room for the birth.

Preparing for a home birth

There are some useful ways you can make your home birth comfortable for yourself and convenient for the midwife.

☐ Make sure your bed is firm so that you have something to push against and can avoid getting a puddle of amniotic fluid under your hips. If necessary put a board under the mattress. You may decide not to use the bed, but do have it ready so that all your options are open.

☐ The most convenient way to make the bed is as follows. Make it up with fresh sheets. Put on a plastic sheet (an old shower curtain will do) and cover with clean, old linens. In this way the old sheets and plastic can be taken off after the birth, leaving you in a freshly made bed.

☐ Collect newspapers for several weeks before your due date. You can lay these on the floor to make a path from bathroom to bed to catch any drips. Newsprint is considered clean and inhibits the growth of germs so, if you don't object, newspaper can be put underneath you as a bed pan.

☐ Prepare a work area, such as a table top or a dressing-table, that is within easy reach of the bed for supplies.

EQUIPMENT FOR A HOME BIRTH

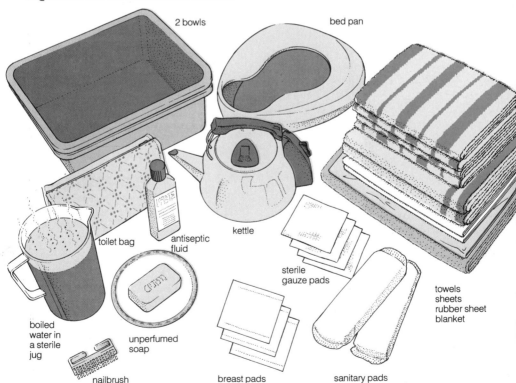

2 bowls

bed pan

toilet bag

antiseptic fluid

kettle

sterile gauze pads

towels
sheets
rubber sheet
blanket

boiled water in a sterile jug

unperfumed soap

nailbrush

breast pads

sanitary pads

AIDS FOR LABOR

Your partner or birth assistant will also need to pack a small bag with aids for the labor. Prepare and take with you a bag containing:
- a small natural sponge to moisten her mouth
- lipsalve or vaseline to prevent her lips becoming chapped
- frozen picnic freezing pack or hot-water bottle to put against her back if she has bad backache
- a thermos of diluted fruit juice or water (check if the hospital allows) for her to sip during labor
- drinks and sandwiches for yourself, but enough left over for her if after delivery she's just missed a meal
- books, playing cards, scrabble, jigsaws, cassette deck and tapes to occupy you both while you're waiting between contractions
- coins for the hospital phone
- leg warmers or thick socks if she starts to shake during the later stages
- washcloth to mop her face if she becomes too hot

☐ Have a couch or a comfortable chair for your attendant to lie down and have a rest on during the labor.

☐ Clear a large area if you plan to have a mobile labor. Have some freshly ironed sheets nearby if you want to deliver onto the floor.

☐ To prepare yourself you should have a bath, or, if the waters have broken a shower in case of infection. Otherwise, wash your hands to beyond the wrists, wash your thighs 12in down either side, and wash the pubic area, all with antiseptic soap and dry with a clean towel, sterile cloth or gauze pad. Make sure that you make one clean motion from the top downwards from your vagina to thighs.

☐ Have ready a clean nightgown, sanitary pads and underpants for yourself, and a large blanket, a disposable diaper and a nightgown or stretch suit for the baby. Prepare the crib with the baby's bedding and blankets in place.

What to take to the hospital

Several weeks before your baby is due, pack your hospital case with all the things you will need for your stay there. Ask the hospital if they provide a clothes list. Most hospitals provide diapers and all the baby's clothing during your stay, but check in advance. The baby will therefore only need the clothes and blankets to come home in. Your partner can bring these in after the birth, but leave them packed up with your own coming-home clothes. Remember to set aside something as loose fitting as your maternity clothes for yourself. Your breasts will have increased in size when the milk comes in and your abdomen won't have gone down.

For you
- 2–3 nightgowns opening down the front if you plan to breastfeed
- 2–3 nursing bras (see p. 125)
- breast pads
- bathrobe
- slippers
- 4 pairs of underpants
- sanitary pads, the stick-on ones are best; buy the super absorbent for the first days
- toilet bag and contents – including toothbrush, deodorant etc.
- tissues or a soft toilet roll
- make-up, face and hand cream and shampoo
- mirror
- coins for the telephone

For the baby
- 2 diapers
- undershirt
- stretch suit or nightgown
- shawl
- bonnet
- cotton receiving blanket

157

ARRANGEMENTS FOR YOUR OTHER CHILDREN

If you have a family, every member should be involved in your pregnancy. Children should be informed about what is going on and how the pregnancy is progressing, according to their age and how much information they can absorb and understand. Even a very young child will notice that your abdomen is swelling and will want to know why. Give an honest and accurate answer and let your child feel the baby kicking inside you. If your child or children are old enough, put a chart up on the wall of what happens to you and the baby in pregnancy and follow it through as your pregnancy progresses.

If you are having a home birth you must decide whether you want your children to be involved or not. Although it may seem sensible not to restrict the child if he follows your pregnancy through, the experience could be a frightening one. If you decide to involve him, don't be surprised if he gets bored and wants to go off and play. Someone responsible must be there, besides your partner, to take care of him during the labor. Run through everything with him ahead of time, especially the birth of the placenta, which is often the bloodiest part. Warn him that you won't be able to answer his questions because you'll be busy, and that if the nurse-midwife asks him to leave the room, he must do exactly as she says.

If you are going into the hospital, explain to your child what is going to happen and what arrangements will be made, as long as he is old enough to understand. Even if you plan to be in the hospital for a short time, say 24 or 48 hours, you will have to make arrangements for someone to take care of your child. If you possibly can, make sure

Chart the progress of your pregnancy with your other children and involve them with it as much as possible.

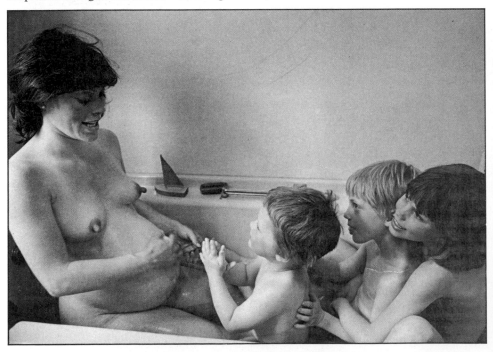

that he goes to a familiar place, to someone he knows and likes. If this isn't possible, gradually introduce your child to any new surroundings and the new person well in advance of your going into the hospital to have your baby.

Make sure that your child knows exactly how long you will be apart. Prepare him in other ways by pointing out small babies to him, showing him pictures of his babyhood and relate this to the coming arrival. Buy him a doll of his own so that he feels he has a baby too. It helps too if your partner increases his involvement with the child, particularly with the usual routines of bathing, feeding and storytime.

If you have a baby it is fairly easy for you to make arrangements for him to be looked after while you are giving birth. But if your child is older I think it helps a great deal if you act out rehearsals. Compile a timetable of what you will do when labor starts. Go over this in detail with your child so that he becomes familiar with the future events. If you rehearse the whole scheme together several times he will feel happy and secure in the knowledge that you are taking special care of him. One day, well before you expect the baby, you might like to go through the whole plan and act it out from the beginning to the end. "Now this morning we are going to try out what we will do on the day or night that Mommy is going to have the baby in the hospital. First of all we will get your suitcase, which we packed last week with all your clothes and toys and your favorite book. Then you'll put your coat on, get into the car and go over to granny's ... etc."

WHEN LABOR STARTS
Home birth
1 Call the midwife.
2 Call your partner or birth assistant.
3 Contact whoever is caring for your other children and alert them.
4 Check that the room is ready.
5 Have a hot bath or shower.

Hospital birth
1 Call your doctor and confer with him or her. If it is time to be admitted, call an ambulance if you are not being driven to the hospital.
2 Call your partner or birth assistant.
3 Alert whoever is caring for your children that you will be going in to the hospital soon.
4 Get the suitcase and your coat and handbag.
5 Sit down and wait for your partner or the ambulance.

If someone is driving you to the hospital, you should know how to get there and how long it will take. Plot an alternative route in case the traffic is heavy or you find the road blocked for some reason. Whenever possible choose well-made roads so that your journey will be comfortable. Find out which hospital entrance you should use, during the day and night, so that you reach the delivery room quickly. Make sure that you and the driver are thoroughly familiar with all this information; if it puts your mind at rest, do a trial run.

In the week or two before you go into labor there may be signs that something is about to happen.
1 One of the earliest signs is lightening or engagement, when the baby's head drops into your pelvis.
2 The baby's engagement causes an increase in pressure on the bladder and you will find that you want to pass urine more frequently again.
3 Braxton Hicks contractions become more frequent and may get stronger.
4 Often vaginal secretions increase a day or so before labor starts.
5 You may notice a slight weight loss in the last week.
6 Some women experience a nesting instinct; they feel driven to clean and straighten the house.

159

15 Labor and birth

This is the culmination of your pregnancy – the high point to which all your preparations have been leading. You will be hoping for a pleasurable labor, not necessarily pain free – that would be unrealistic – but a relaxed and happy one.

You will be happy, despite the discomfort, if everything and everyone around you is known to you. You will be relaxed if you understand what is happening to you and are confident that you can control your body and help during the delivery. If you learn about labor and birth and practice the exercises and breathing techniques you should feel less pain and be alert so that you can enjoy giving birth.

LABOR

Labor can be divided into well-defined stages. There is a stage before labor begins, sometimes called pre-labor (see opposite). The first stage of labor can be divided into two; the early phase is the time when you start going into labor and when contractions may be short, irregular and not too painful. This culminates in the late first stage of labor and transition when your contractions become regular, more frequent, painful and result in full dilation of the cervix. The second stage of labor is when you push the baby through the birth canal; it ends with the birth of your baby. Labor is not complete until you have gone through the third stage, which is delivery of the placenta (afterbirth).

Pain in labor

Every woman feels the pain of contractions differently but in early labor they may be similar to menstrual cramps; sometimes they're confined to mild backache. The kind of labor that proceeds well into the first stage with nothing more than gradually worsening backache is often called a back labor (see p. 169). Very often a contraction feels like a wave of discomfort right across your abdomen that reaches a crescendo for a few seconds and then diminishes. At the same time you can feel a hardening and tightening of the uterine muscle, which is held at the peak of its intensity for a few seconds until the muscle begins to relax. You have absolutely no control over your contractions – they are "involuntary" – though your state of mind during labor can have a profound effect on whether you perceive them as more or less painful. Most women assume that contractions will get longer, more frequent and stronger in a steady pattern. This is not so – don't be disturbed if your contractions seem to vary. It is absolutely normal for a strong contraction, for example, to be followed by a weaker one that doesn't last quite as long. It is also normal for the contractions to follow one another relentlessly – this is more likely if your labor has been induced and is kept going with an intravenous drip (see p. 188).

Onset of labor

Most people think that the onset of labor will be very clear; pains will come, contractions will start and you'll know. It often isn't clear at all. Three things might happen, though they don't necessarily mean that birth is imminent.

☐ The blood-tinged, gelatinous plug of mucus that has blocked the cervical canal during pregnancy can be dislodged during the early first stage of labor if not before and always precedes rupture of the membranes. It is sometimes called the show and means that the cervix is beginning to stretch.

☐ Your membranes may rupture at any time up to the delivery. Leakage of the amniotic fluid varies from woman to woman. In some it's a gush and in others it's just a slight dribble that can be stemmed by wearing a sanitary pad. There is no pain accompanying rupture of the membranes and the flow depends on the site, size of the break and whether or not the baby's head can plug the hole. Even though the membranes have ruptured you can continue your usual routine though

LENGTH OF LABOR

This is usually longest with a first baby, an average 12–14 hours. Thereafter labor lasts an average seven hours. In general terms the lighter the contractions, the longer the labor will be. A fast labor tends to start with long, slow contractions and proceeds in the same way.

you should contact your doctor or the hospital immediately.

☐ You may feel a dull backache or if you have experienced Braxton Hicks contractions during the third trimester you may mistake the early contractions of your labor for stronger Braxton Hicks. Severe Braxton Hicks contractions can be mistaken for labor, however, and this is known as a "false labor."

Time these early contractions over an hour and if they get closer together and longer in duration, you're probably in labor. Contractions, once it's established that you're in labor, are timed from the beginning of one to the beginning of the next. They tend to be 30 to 60 seconds long at first, building up to 75 seconds in length during the most active phase of labor.

THE PRESENTATION

The presenting part of your baby is the part that will be born first. Most babies lie in a well-flexed (curled up) position with knees bent, arms and legs crossed and chin resting on the chest (near right). The way the baby is presenting can affect your labor and birth; for example, a posterior presentation (far right) can lead to an erratic back labor (see p. 169). If the head is not well flexed and the face is presenting, labor may be slower and the baby's features may be slightly swollen for about 24 hours.

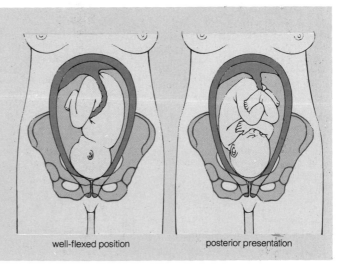

well-flexed position   posterior presentation

Admission to the hospital

When you arrive the nurse will prepare you for the birth.

● She will ask you questions about the labor so far – whether your waters have broken, how frequently the contractions are coming and whether you have moved your bowels.

● You will be asked to undress and get into a hospital gown.

● You will then be examined; a nurse or doctor will palpate your abdomen to feel the baby's position, will listen to the fetal heartbeat, take your blood pressure, pulse and temperature and give you an internal examination to see how far your cervix has dilated.

● You will be asked to give a urine sample to test for protein and sugar.

● You may then be shaved unless you ask not to be (see p. 51).

● If you haven't moved your bowels recently, you may be given an enema or suppository (see p. 51)

● You are then taken to the labor room. If you have any questions or you want to make your feelings known to the staff, now is the time to mention your preferences and how you want your labor managed if all goes well.

The fetal heartbeat will be constantly monitored either with a fetoscope or with electronic monitors (see p. 190).

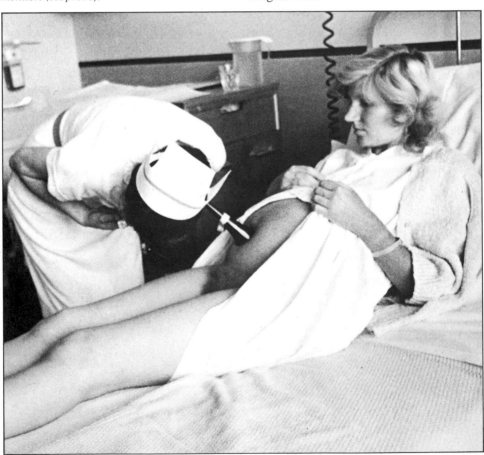

BREATHING FOR LABOR AND BIRTH

If you have learnt a breathing and relaxation technique (see pp. 131–2) during your pregnancy, now is the time to put it into practice. Your birth assistant can help by tapping out a rhythm or using words like "breath," "breath," "steady," "steady" to help you to concentrate. The pattern may have a greater effect if you can maintain eye contact with your birth assistant.

Early first stage

The contractions will be gentle and you should be able to breathe deeply and evenly throughout. Practice a welcoming response to a contraction by trying not to tense up. Greet each one with a slow, even breath out.

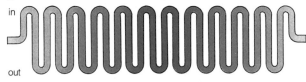

in
out
even breathing
length of contraction

Late first stage

Take your opening breath out and then try to breathe above the contractions; light, short breaths that hardly seem to involve the lower parts of your body at all. Take a deep breath and relax when it is all over to signal to yourself and those around you that the contraction is over.

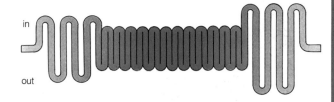

in
out
slow breathing   light breathing   deep breaths
length of contraction

Transitional stage

Try the shallowest breathing of all – panting – though without hyperventilating and starving your body of carbon dioxide. Breathe only in your mouth. If you feel dizzy, your birth assistant can cup his hands over your nose and mouth while you are breathing.

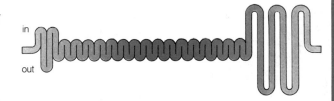

in
out
light breaths   panting   deep even breathing
length of contraction

Second stage

This should be the most natural pattern of breathing for you. Take a deep breath and hold it while bearing down and letting your pelvic floor bulge outward. Let your push be long and smooth. Then repeat if the contraction is still intense and lie back slowly and gently when it ends.

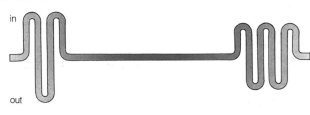

in
out
deep breath   pushing   even breathing
length of contraction

THE FIRST STAGE OF LABOR

This is when the cervix opens out (dilates) fully to allow the baby's head to pass through. Before it can dilate, the normally thick, fairly tough cervix becomes thinned and softened and is gradually pulled up by the contracting uterine muscle. This is known as effacement. The muscle of the upper segment of the uterus contracts and exerts pressure on the lower segment, which in turn transmits the pull of the contractions to the cervix. As a result, once the cervix has stretched, it begins to dilate with each contraction until the entire cervical canal is eliminated. You are then fully dilated. The degrees of dilation of the cervix have been standardized, so that it can be described accurately and progress charted. If you ask your doctor how labor is progressing, he or she will nearly always respond in terms of the number of centimeters of cervical dilation or perhaps with the number of fingers (one finger is approximately one centimeter).

Dilation is normally given in one centimeter increments. At five or six centimeters the cervix is described as being half dilated. When the cervix is said to be fully dilated it is approximately 10 centimeters in diameter. This is the completion of the first stage of labor though in real terms the first stage moves gradually and smoothly through a transitional stage and into the second stage without punctuation.

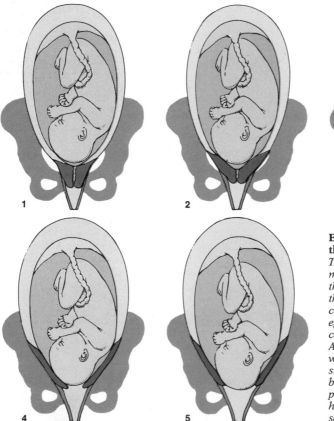

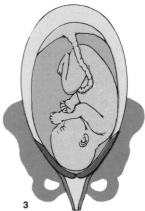

Effacement and dilation of the cervix
The normally tough cervix (1) must be thinned out (2) before the baby's head can pass through. When the cervical canal is eliminated – fully effaced (3) – further contractions dilate the cervix. At seven centimeters the doctor will feel only the front and the sides of the cervix around the baby's head (4). When the last part of the cervix at the front has disappeared (5) you are said to be fully dilated.

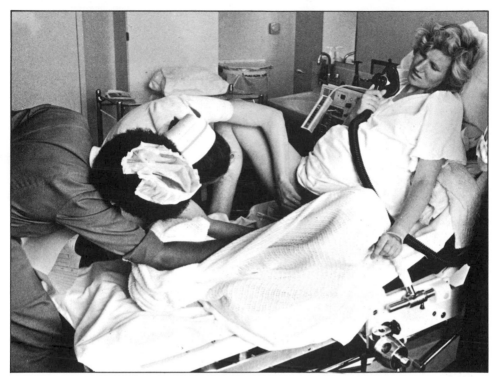

Examinations during labor

After the admission procedure, the anesthesiologist will visit you if you want some form of pain relief (see p. 182). If not, you will be left with your partner or birth assistant and a nurse or midwife will be with you throughout your labor.

The fetal heart will be constantly monitored either by fetoscope or a machine (see p. 190). Internal examinations will be done periodically (about every two hours) to check on cervical effacement and dilation. This is usually done with you lying flat on your back. If this proves to be an uncomfortable position for you, ask if it can be done with you lying on your side.

Each time you have an internal examination ask the medical attendant how you are progressing. If you've never before met the person who comes to examine you and they don't introduce themselves, ask who they are and what

Sometimes internal examinations can be painful, so try to relax during them.

they are going to do and introduce yourself. If you feel that your contractions are getting longer and stronger and you haven't had an internal examination for a while, then ask for one. It is quite cheering to find that your cervical dilation has progressed between examinations.

It is possible that your assistant or companion will be asked to leave during your preparation and any internal examinations. This is absolutely unnecessary and people who have nothing to do with your birth will be coming into the delivery room all the time – so make sure that your companion stays.

You may be asked questions during an internal examination or while you are having a contraction. Concentrate on what you are doing and answer the question when the contraction is over.

165

ADVICE TO BIRTH ASSISTANT

● During pre-labor, encourage her to sleep and to conserve her strength. You may see a burst of energy which is the nesting instinct, but do tell her firmly to rest and put her feet up.

● In the early stages of labor and if the membranes haven't ruptured, encourage her to take a warm bath and help her to get in and out of the tub so that she doesn't slip. If they have ruptured, a shower is best (see p. 157).

● Unless she is feeling nauseous encourage her to eat and drink lightly. Natural fruit juice and honey contain sugars which will give her plenty of energy. You should eat something too.

● When the contractions begin you should time them and note the interval between them (from the start of one to the beginning of another) and how long each contraction lasts. Put your hand on her abdomen so that you can feel the peak of the contraction.

● One of your most important roles is to coach her through the contractions, giving comfort and support. Never criticize, use positive words and praise as much as you can. Don't be offended if she turns away from you and seeks reassurance from the medical staff who are experienced in childbirth. She is not rejecting you.

● It is very soothing to wipe her face, massage her back or her abdomen or just hold hands.

● Be on the watch for any signs of tension in her neck, shoulders and forehead and remind her to relax and how to do it. It's a good idea for her to keep her mouth loose between contractions, so if you see any signs of tension encourage her to close her mouth and drop her jaw.

● If she is up and mobile remind her to empty her bladder every hour. Whenever she does get up and move about, stay near her because any kind of activity can increase the contractions. Go with her to the bathroom; your presence outside the door can be reassuring.

● Observe her moods and fit in with them. If she wants to stay quiet, then do so, but if she wants to be distracted, play a game of cards or scrabble.

● When you arrive at the hospital and she is having contractions, simply sign the essential forms and go directly to the labor ward. Any other forms can be filled out later. The most important priority is to move her as little as possible and get her settled as comfortably and as quickly as you can. Try to prevent anything in the hospital from making her anxious or distracting from her control of her labor.

● If the staff insist that you go to a father's waiting room while she is "prepared," stay there for about 20 or 30 minutes and then go back to the labor ward. Identify yourself to the first nurse you see and ask to be allowed to join your partner.

● When drugs are offered make sure that she knows what the drugs are for. If she feels like trying to hang on, help her to do so but remember that there is absolutely no reason why she should not be given drugs if they are medically indicated in her case.

● If you're at home, the midwife will probably be on her own for most of the time, so be ready to assist whenever she asks. Do as she says quickly.

● When labor is well established, you could place your hand on her abdomen so that you can feel it begin to tighten and know when the next contraction is coming. As the uterus starts to harden and rise tell her to take in a deep breath. You can make sure that she is not caught off-guard by contractions and therefore she will be able to control them better.

Touching and stroking at any time during labor can be immensely helpful.

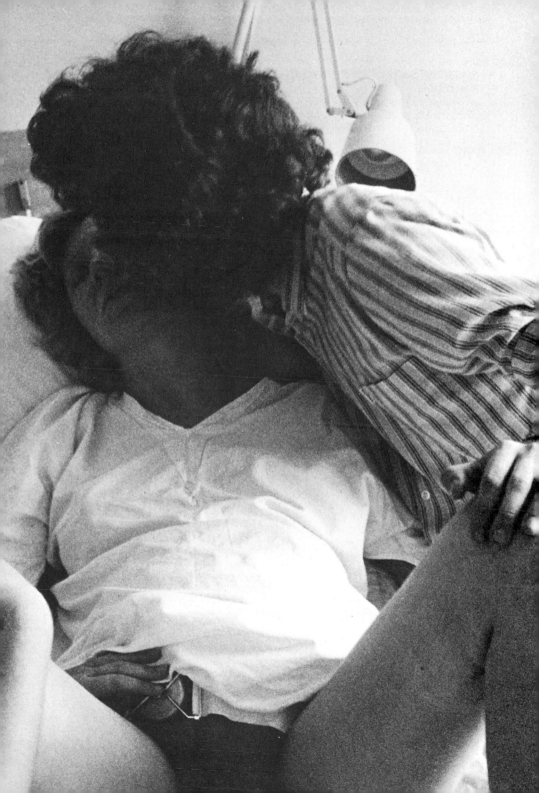

POSITIONS FOR THE FIRST STAGE

None of these positions is right or wrong; you have to find the most comfortable position for you. Move around and keep trying new ones. Use the furniture or your partner as an aid. Many women like to move around and when the contraction starts, take up the chosen position.

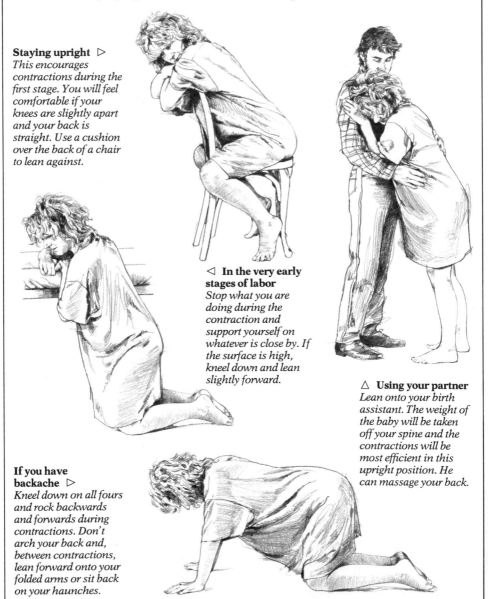

Staying upright ▷
This encourages contractions during the first stage. You will feel comfortable if your knees are slightly apart and your back is straight. Use a cushion over the back of a chair to lean against.

◁ **In the very early stages of labor**
Stop what you are doing during the contraction and support yourself on whatever is close by. If the surface is high, kneel down and lean slightly forward.

△ **Using your partner**
Lean onto your birth assistant. The weight of the baby will be taken off your spine and the contractions will be most efficient in this upright position. He can massage your back.

If you have backache ▷
Kneel down on all fours and rock backwards and forwards during contractions. Don't arch your back and, between contractions, lean forward onto your folded arms or sit back on your haunches.

The Transitional stage

This is the stage from the end of the first stage to the beginning of the second stage of labor. It is the shortest stage of labor, averaging about one hour, often 30 minutes or less, but it can be quite hard to cope with. After several hours in the first stage, some women become discouraged and feel that they can't go on without some pain relief. There may be some shaking and shivering which is physiological and not abnormal or anything to be afraid of. Simply because of all the hormone changes that are going on you may feel some irritability and ill-temper. Some women feel so nauseated and they want to vomit. Don't resist this urge because you will feel a lot better afterwards. There is usually some excitement and restlessness, and every position seems uncomfortable. You may feel some anxiety for your own safety and for the baby's, and you may feel sleepy between contractions because most of the oxygen in your body is being taken up by the uterus and the baby and your brain is relatively short of it.

Some women feel the urge to push during this stage but don't bear down until an internal examination confirms that your cervix is fully dilated. If you feel a strong urge to push but it is too soon to do so, use the panting and blowing breathing technique (see p. 132) until the doctor tells you it is safe to start to push.

ADVICE TO BIRTH ASSISTANT

- Try to get her to relax, refrain from asking questions and remove perspiration if she's sweating a lot.
- If she tells you not to touch her, refrain but stay near the bed. If she feels sick and wants to vomit, get a basin and encourage her to do so. Always praise her.
- If her legs start to tremble, put on her socks and hold her legs firmly.
- If you notice that she is beginning to grunt and make pushing movements inform the nurse immediately. This is a difficult stage, and you should perhaps tell her that you think she is in transition and the baby will be born soon.
- You will know that the delivery is imminent when the doctor says that the head is crowning – it is beginning to emerge from the vaginal opening.

For most women the end of the transition stage is marked by a noticeable change in the pattern of breathing, you may grunt involuntarily, and this is because you will start to feel the urge to bear down. The need to push becomes very strong. Do tell your assistant to alert the staff that you are ready to push. They will confirm that the cervix has dilated 10 centimeters and the second stage is beginning. Your baby is about to be born.

BACK LABOR

If your baby is in the posterior position, its head may be pressing against your sacrum. This usually results in a long, erratic labor accompanied by backache. In this position the baby's head is not properly flexed and a larger diameter presents. However, the baby usually rotates before passing through the birth canal and the birth itself is normal. If your backache is particularly bad, there are ways to relieve it.

- Keep moving, and during contractions take up a position in which the pressure is taken off your back; for example on all fours, leaning into a chair, or rocking to and fro.
- Nullify the pressure with counter pressure. Your birth assistant can apply pressure with fists or something round such as a tennis ball against your back.
- Apply a hot water bottle to the lower part of your back between contractions.
- Don't lie flat on your back; the baby's head then presses onto your spine.
- Massage the buttocks and the lower back (see p. 133).

POSITIONS DURING TRANSITION

This is a difficult stage in which to find a comfortable position. Contractions seem relentless, but if you understand that the baby will be born soon, that should give you the confidence to stay calm and patient. You probably won't feel like moving around so much but try to change positions now and again.

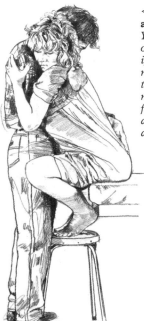

◁ **Using your birth assistant**
You can lean forward onto your partner, and if you are on a high narrow hospital bed, this will make you feel more secure. Put your feet on a stool or chair, and keep your knees apart.

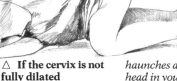

△ **If the cervix is not fully dilated**
If you feel the need to bear down, use gravity to slow the baby down while the cervix continues to dilate. Kneel down and either sit back on your haunches and rest your head in your arms against a low chair, or lean forward and put your head on your arms on the floor and your bottom in the air. This takes pressure off the lower back.

▽ **If you want to rest**
Lie down on your side with cushions under your head and upper thigh. Keep your legs as wide apart as possible.

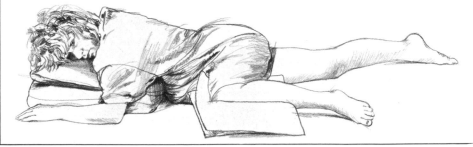

POSITIONS FOR DELIVERY

You will know by now from your experience of labor what position you want to give birth in. Take advice from your medical attendants; they will coach you through the pushing stage. Enjoy yourself and take your time.

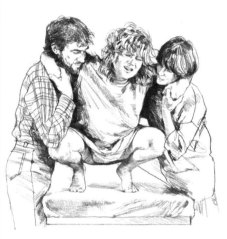

◁ **Squatting**
This opens up the pelvis, relaxes the pelvic floor and vaginal opening and uses the force of gravity to deliver the baby. To squat on a bed, you will need two helpers to support you so that you feel safe.

Supported squat ▷
Your partner can support you by taking your weight on his arms. He should keep his back straight, and his knees slightly bent.

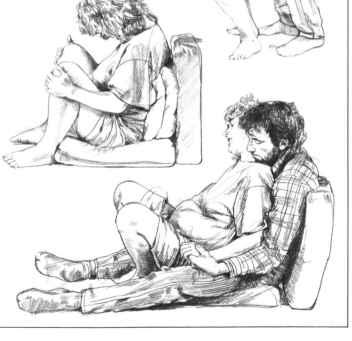

A common delivery position ▷
Sit propped up with cushions, hold onto your knees and drop your chin on your chest. You can lie back and relax between each contraction and conserve your energy. You will be able to see the baby emerge in this position.

Semi-upright position ▷
If you feel happier being close to your partner during the delivery, you can lean back against him. His closeness will give you confidence and he can encourage you to push during contractions.

THE SECOND STAGE

For a first baby the second stage generally doesn't last longer than two hours – the average is around one hour – and it may be as little as 15 to 20 minutes for subsequent babies. Bearing down is a reflex, an instinctive urge to push down which is caused by the baby's head pressing on the pelvic floor and the rectum. Even if you know nothing about the mechanics of labor you will know

ADVICE TO BIRTH ASSISTANT

● Remind her to relax her pelvic floor during pushing. She should take two or three deep breaths and push her hardest at the peak of contractions. She should push in a strong, steady way.

● Remind her to look in the mirror so that she can see the baby emerging.

● If you are in the hospital and are asked to leave the delivery room suddenly, do so without question. There may be a medical emergency and staff will have to move very fast. You cannot guarantee that you will not be in the way. Leave the delivery room but stay close by outside.

● Remind her to lie back and relax fully between contractions so that she conserves her strength for pushing.

● You are now more of an observer once the baby's head has crowned. The doctor will be the one who coaches your partner through the pushing stage.

● Don't expect your partner to communicate with you during the birth. She will be preoccupied and may not notice you for some time.

● When the baby is placed on her stomach, if possible put your arms around them both to keep them warm and signal that you're still there.

● Be ready for your own and your partner's reactions – tears, silence, whoops of joy, perhaps even squeamishness on your part. It's all perfectly normal and understandable.

automatically to take a deep breath, so lowering your diaphragm which exerts pressure on the uterus and helps the pushing. You then hold your breath, slightly bend your knees and strain downwards. Pushing is painless for you and doesn't hurt the baby but it is still quite hard work, much harder work if you are lying on your back because you actually have to push the baby uphill (see p. 52) and less hard if you are in a semi-upright position (see p. 171) and have the force of gravity helping you. Your pushing should be smooth and continuous. All of the muscular effort should be down and out. It should be fairly slow and gradual so that the vaginal tissues and muscles are given time to stretch and accommodate your baby's head without tearing or making an episiotomy necessary.

You should push during a contraction. Your pushing effort only *helps* the uterus to expel the baby. The involuntary muscles of the uterus can expel the baby on their own. So you help most by beginning your pushing effort with the peak intensity of each contraction.

During pushing, the pelvic floor and the anal area should be fully relaxed, so make a conscious effort to relax this part of your body (see p. 113). You may lose a little stool but don't be embarrassed. Don't worry about urinating either; it is very common. When you've finished a push you will find two slow, deep breaths helpful, but don't relax too quickly at the end of each contraction as the baby will maintain its forward progress if you relax slowly. If you are in the hospital and your labor has been in the labor room so far, it is just before the second stage that you'll be transferred to the delivery room and delivered on a delivery table unless you've made alternative arrangements with the hospital (see p. 54).

Pushing is instinctive. Even if you don't understand why, you will automatically take a deep breath and push downwards.

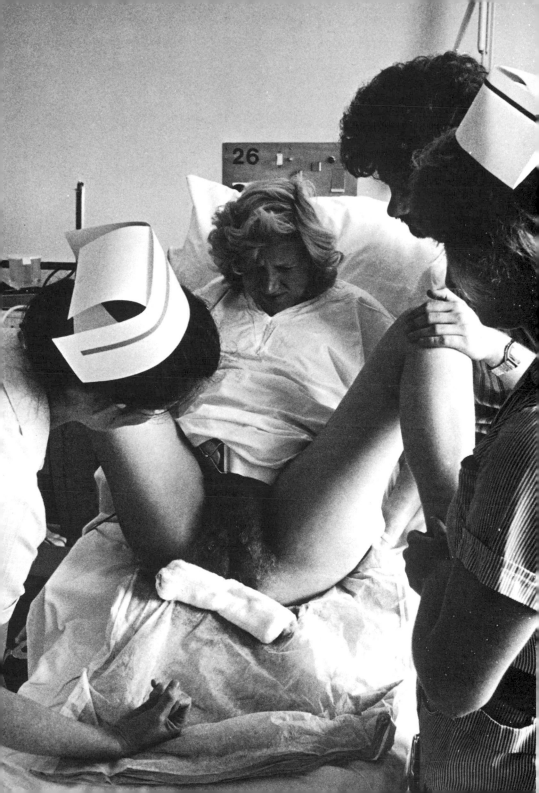

Birth

The first sign that the baby is coming is bulging of the anus and perineum. With each contraction more and more of the baby's head appears at the vaginal opening, though it may slip back slightly between contractions. If you're watching in a mirror don't be disheartened, this is normal. After crowning, the head will be delivered in the next contraction or two. You can reach down at this point and touch the head to reassure yourself.

It is perfectly normal to feel a stinging or burning sensation as the baby stretches the outlet of the birth canal. As soon as you feel it, stop bearing down, pant and allow the uterus to push the baby out on its own. As you stop pushing, lean back and try to go limp. Make a conscious effort to relax the muscles of the perineal floor (see p. 113). The burning or stinging sensation lasts for a short time and is immediately followed by a numb feeling as the baby's head stretches the vaginal tissues so thin that the nerves are blocked, having a natural anesthetic effect. If the medical staff feel you are going to tear badly, this is the moment they may do an episiotomy (see p. 186). They will also check that the cord is not round the baby's neck (see p. 174). As the baby's head is delivered, you will feel a sensation like toothpaste coming out of a tube.

When the head is delivered, the baby's back is uppermost and it's face is pointing towards your rectum. Almost immediately, however, the baby will start to rotate its shoulders so that it is facing your right or left thigh. The direction depends on the baby's position in the uterus. The doctor will wipe its eyes, nose and mouth with clean gauze, and remove any fluid from the nose and upper air passages. Now there's a breathing space when the uterine contractions stop for a few minutes. When they restart, it's hardly necessary for you to push because the first uterine contraction is usually sufficient to deliver first one shoulder and the next contraction will deliver the other and the rest of your baby will slide out.

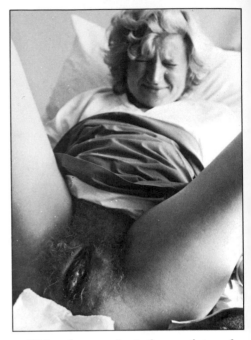

1 *With each contraction in the second stage of labor, more of the baby's head appears at the vaginal opening. The anus and the perineum bulge out with the pressure of the head.*

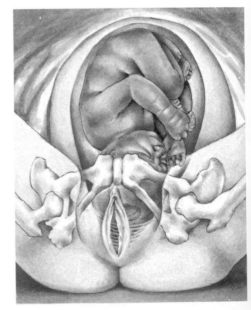

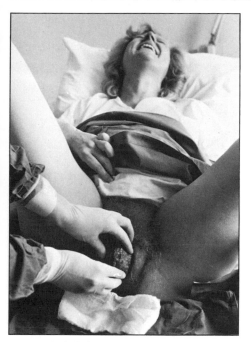

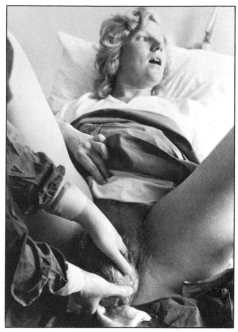

2 *As the baby's head crowns, the stinging sensation is followed by numbness as the vaginal tissues are stretched so thin that the nerves are blocked. The head slips out at last.*

3 *The head is born facing downwards towards the rectum but the baby immediately turns to face your thigh to get into a good position for the birth of the body.*

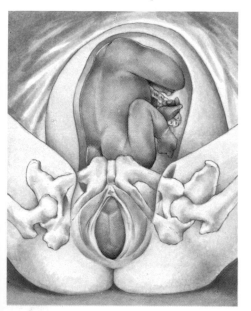

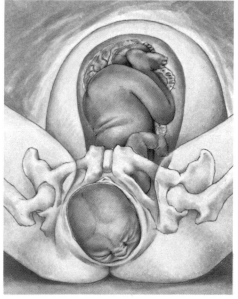

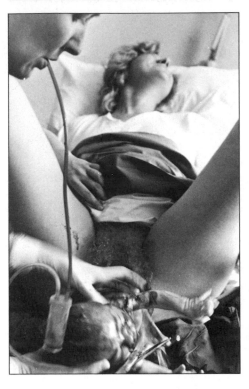

4 *The nurse will clear any fluid from the baby's air passages. The next uterine contraction is usually sufficient to deliver the body.*

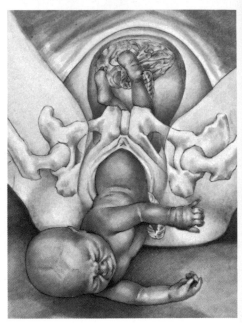

The doctor usually assists this last part of the delivery by putting thumbs and fingers under the armpits of your baby and lifting her upwards towards your abdomen. If you're feeling alert and you're in a position to do so, you can bend down, and pull your baby out for yourself and on to your abdomen.

Your baby may cry first when delivered and will be crying lustily a few seconds after birth. If the breathing is normal, there's absolutely no reason why you should not take hold of the baby immediately. Ask if you can lay the baby on your abdomen and keep her warm with your arms and those of your partner. If there's a danger of the baby being cold, all three of you can be kept warm with a warm towel or blanket. Your gentle stroking movements, your soothing voice and the sound of your heartbeat are all right for your baby.

Your baby will probably be a bluish color at first and may be covered with the white greasy vernix (see p. 74). She will have streaks of blood on her head and body and depending on your delivery her head may be elongated after the journey down the birth canal. The doctor will make a check of her general condition (see p. 206). If there is fluid in the mouth or nose or air passages, the doctor or nurse will want to make sure that it's cleared and breathing is normal. He or she will suck it out again. If the baby doesn't start to breathe immediately, the doctor will take her and give her oxygen. Don't be alarmed at the sudden activity. As soon as the baby's breathing is normal, she will be returned to you to hold.

5 *The baby is born and handed to the mother while the cord is clamped and eventually cut. The uterus will soon begin to contract again after about 10–15 minutes to expel the placenta. This is not usually painful.*

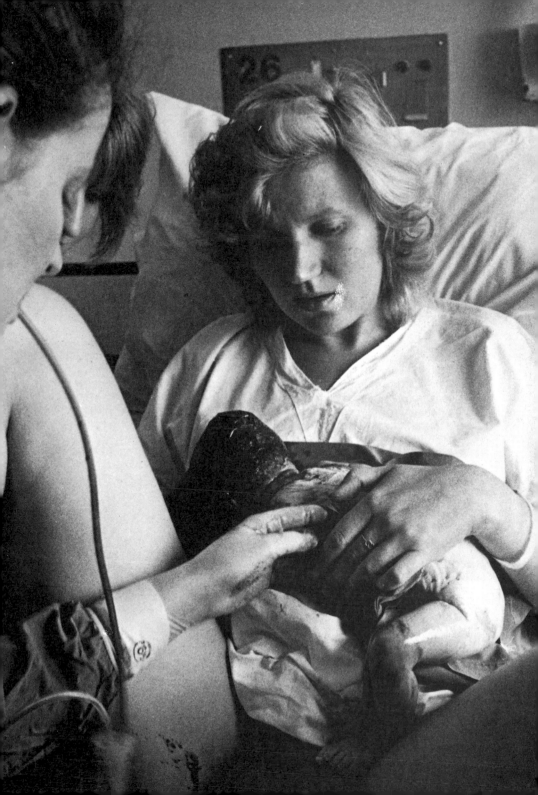

THIRD STAGE

When the baby is born the uterus rests and after about 15 minutes starts to contract comparatively painlessly again to expel the placenta. This is the third stage of labor. You may find that you are so involved with your baby that you hardly notice this stage. For some women, however, the delivery of the placenta is painful enough to require continued breathing and relaxation techniques. Oxytocin is naturally produced in response to seeing and touching your baby, but most of all putting her to the breast to feed; it increases the contractions of the uterus and helps to expel the placenta more quickly.

What is happening during the third stage of labor is detachment of the placenta from the uterine wall. The large blood vessels, about the thickness of a pencil, that run to and from the placenta, are simply torn across. The reason why most women do not bleed is that the muscle fibers of the uterus are arranged in a criss-cross fashion, and when the uterus contracts down the muscles tighten around the blood vessels, preventing them from bleeding. This is why it's absolutely essential that the uterus contracts down into a hard ball once the placenta has been expelled. The uterus can be kept tightly contracted by massaging it intermittently for an hour or so after the third stage is complete.

The placenta slips out with a gentle squelch. It looks rather like a piece of liver and many women and their partners like to look at it and examine it. It is an amazing organ – it has been the life-support system for your baby for nine months. Once the placenta is delivered it's examined to make sure that it's complete and none of it has been left behind. If any of the placenta has been retained by the uterus it can be a cause of hemorrhage later on (see p. 198).

Shivering and shaking can be quite profound after delivery of the placenta. After delivery of my second child I was shivering so much and my teeth were chattering so that I couldn't speak and couldn't breathe properly. My own explanation for this reaction is that for nine months I had a little furnace inside me, producing quite a lot of heat, and my body had adjusted to take account of that heat production by turning my own thermostat down slightly. When my baby left my body, I was deprived of that heat and the drop of body temperature was probably a few degrees. The only way the body can raise its temperature is to generate heat through muscular work. That's exactly what shivering does: by rapid contraction and relaxation of muscles, heat is produced. The shivering usually passes in about half an hour, during which time the body temperature has been brought back up to normal and your own thermostat reset. Often the muscles in the legs feel quite sore for a day or two. Take long socks or leg

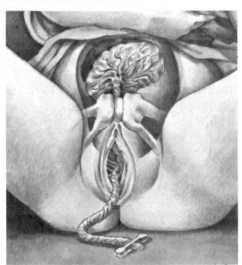

When the contractions resume, they will be less painful. One or two pushes should expel the placenta. The midwife will put one hand on your uterus and will gently pull on the cord with the other to ease the placenta carefully out. It is important that no part of the placenta is left behind (see p. 198).

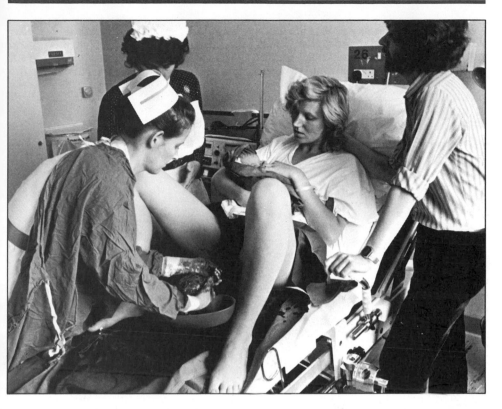

warmers into the delivery room to keep you warm and reduce muscle strain.

Clamping the cord

There is no need for the unseemly rush to clamp the cord that there used to be 20 years ago when I first qualified. It's generally believed that the baby benefits from the return of placental blood through the umbilical cord and that it should not be clamped until it stops pulsating. When the time is right, the cord is divided between a pair of clamps placed 5–6in from the baby's navel. (Blood can flow from the placenta to the baby only if the baby is at a lower level than the uterus.) The cord will need to be clamped and cut if it is looped tightly around the baby's neck. This is quite common, and the baby will then be delivered very quickly. Usually the midwife will be able to slip the cord out from around the baby's head and

You can hold your baby during the third stage of labor when the placenta is expelled.

the delivery can proceed without immediate clamping.

Now you should be left alone, in the warmth of your house or the hospital delivery room. You can feed your baby and relax after your hard work. If you have chosen not to breastfeed, don't worry, your baby won't be hungry. Just concentrate on getting to know her and learn to recognize her face. If you are in the hospital, ask the staff to leave. They should welcome the break and if all is well you should be left alone. You will presently be washed down, stitched if necessary and asked to pass urine to check that everything is working all right. You can change into your own nightgown. The nurse will wipe the baby and weigh her and put her in the crib ready for transferral to the postnatal ward.

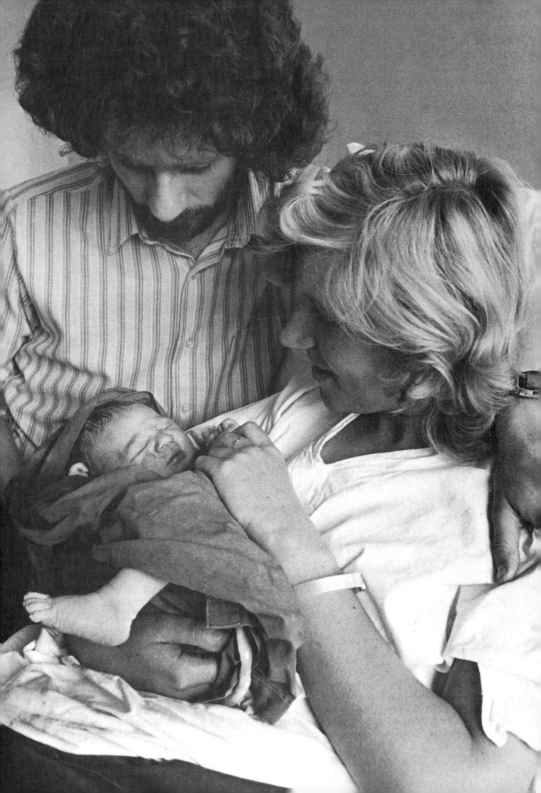

Your baby is born and all the things you thought you'd do and say seem to be lost in the wonder of this little human being, complete with perfect features and tiny hands and feet.

Sudden delivery

If you are alone, or if your doctor or midwife has not arrived when the baby is about to be born, try to pant or blow until they arrive. You should be able to keep this up for five minutes even though the urge to push plus the pressure from the baby's head crowning may make it difficult. Whatever you do, don't try to hold your legs together to delay the birth, and don't allow anyone else to do this. If your baby is coming and you cannot comfortably delay it, don't try to interfere. If you are totally alone, sitting on the floor in a semi-upright position is probably the safest and most comfortable one for you to be in. Holding onto something firm with your arms is both sensible and efficient. Make sure that your baby is delivered onto something soft and clean (a sheet, large towel or tablecloth would do). If you can manage you may even help the baby out yourself once the head has been delivered and the shoulders are clear of the vagina. After that sit or lie down with your baby's skin close to your own; your body heat will keep the baby warm. Cover yourselves with a sheet or blanket and put the baby to suckle at your breast while you wait for help to arrive.

Special care neonatal unit

If there is any problem with the baby, such as low birthweight, she may be taken away to the special care neonatal unit. You may feel very disappointed that you can't touch and feed her as you'd planned, but you will find staff sympathetic, so ask to be allowed to help with the care of your baby. Don't panic, ask questions and expect answers that help you to understand what is happening. If you find you can't communicate effectively, ask your partner or a friend to talk to the pediatrician, or nurse in charge. You will be encouraged to breastfeed your baby if you want to even though she is in an incubator. The hospital will supply you with a pump to express your milk for her and it will be fed to her by tube. Touch her as much as you can so that you gain confidence in handling such a tiny baby.

TWINS

Labor is no more painful with a twin delivery than with a single baby. Almost certainly you will be advised to have the babies in the hospital in case you need extra help with the birth if the babies are not presenting properly. There is no reason why your partner shouldn't stay with you during the delivery; discuss the possibility with medical staff in the last trimester. Your doctor will probably recommend an epidural anesthetic (see p. 184) as twin labors can be prolonged or the second baby may have to be turned before delivery.

There is only one first stage if you're having twins. Once the cervix is fully dilated and you're able to push, both babies are pushed out one after the other. There are two second stages, though the second one will be short, especially if the second baby is smaller than the first. The majority of second babies are born within 10–30 minutes of the first.

Emotionally a twin birth is different from a single birth. You'll hardly appreciate the delivery of the second baby, such is the feeling of triumph and joy when the first baby is born. The midwife will examine you to see that the second baby is lying correctly. The contractions will begin again after a few minutes and the membranes will be artificially ruptured. After the second baby is delivered either one or two placentas will be delivered.

PAIN RELIEF IN LABOR

Few labors are painless but stories about the suffering in labor are often exaggerated and distorted, and some women feel that severe pain is so inevitable that it becomes a self-fulfilling prophecy. The amount of pain actually felt almost always bears a strong relationship to what is expected. Of course you should be realistic, but your expectations can be greatly modified by what you learn, the information you are given, and how confident you feel when you go into labor. This is why prenatal classes and breathing exercises which give you the knowledge that you have some control over your body, and therefore some control over pain, are so important to you.

Everyone agrees that fear and ignorance cause tension, stress and anxiety, all of which make pain worse, and may even create pain where there is very little. Information, knowledge and support can go a long way to dispel fear and anxiety, and will also help to ease pain. There's no question that pain can be relieved with drugs, but to my mind the best form of pain relief is information, a calm state of mind and moral support. Armed with these you will find not only that the pain you feel is less, but that you may be strong enough to cope with it without resorting to analgesics or anesthetics which might dim your consciousness and awareness of what's going on – something that most women these days want to avoid.

However, a common practice amongst doctors and midwives is that the pain in childbirth should be relieved. They believe that an important part of their job is to make labor as painfree as possible, and unless asked to refrain may automatically consider the administration of analgesics. This is why it is essential that you discuss pain relief with them during prenatal visits and make your preferences clear (see p. 62) so that you can avoid any misunderstandings and unnecessary tension once your labor has started.

Of course it's impossible to know your own pain threshold in advance and not all problems can be predicted. So it is important to go into labor with an open mind and to accept the pain relief offered if it is considered essential. Whatever happens, don't feel guilty; not everyone has a trouble-free labor and birth.

Decision to accept pain relief

There are two important considerations about the use of painkilling drugs in labor that you should think about. With most drugs, whether they're sedatives which make you feel calm and sleepy, hypnotics which actually send you to sleep, or narcotics which make you feel light-headed and cut off from the normal world, you will lose some of your awareness of what is happening around you. Many women want to experience every second of giving birth and any interference with their level of awareness is unacceptable. The second important factor is that most drugs (but not necessarily anesthetics, there is still research into the possible effects) will cross the placenta to the baby once in the mother's bloodstream, and will be in a higher concentration in the baby's blood than in the mother's blood. Many mothers find this unacceptable. Bearing both of these things in mind, and after getting as much information as you need, make up your mind about your attitude to having painkilling drugs in your labor.

A useful tip is to wait a little while before accepting drugs. Some good news and moral support may be enough to get you over a sticky patch. Ask how far dilated you are, and if you feel that you are making good progress and can hang on, that may increase your resolve. Have a chat with your partner or companion and some encouraging words will give you added strength. So give yourself about 15 minutes after you feel you may want some pain relief before actually having it. During that time you may make quite good progress. You may have even got through the most painful parts of labor and have only a little way to go. You may be astonished at your own strength and resilience and feel that you can manage perfectly well without drugs.

Analgesics

These work by numbing the pain center in the brain. An analgesic can be interpreted as any drug that relieves pain, and therefore would include tranquilizers, sedatives and narcotics. Possible side effects of analgesics are drowsiness, nausea, dizziness, irregular heart rate, and hemorrhage. Because analgesics can lower your blood pressure, they can also slow your labor. Your baby's respiration and behavioral responses may also be affected by a heavy dose of analgesics. One of the most commonly used analgesics in labor is Demerol.

Demerol is a narcotic given by injection in varying dosages during the first stage. It takes about 20 minutes to work and is sometimes combined with other drugs. Demerol relaxes you and relieves your anxiety but its painkilling effect is variable. It is given less frequently than it used to be largely because it was used to relieve maternal fatigue if the first stage of labor was protracted.

With modern aids, mothers no longer become overtired and distressed the way they used to. The safest time to adminster the drug is six to eight hours before delivery. As this is difficult to calculate and the drug wears off in about two hours, it is probably best for those women who are nervous and anxious during the early first stage of labor.

The mask through which you breathe in the gas and air must fit firmly against your face. Used properly it gives a mild level of pain relief.

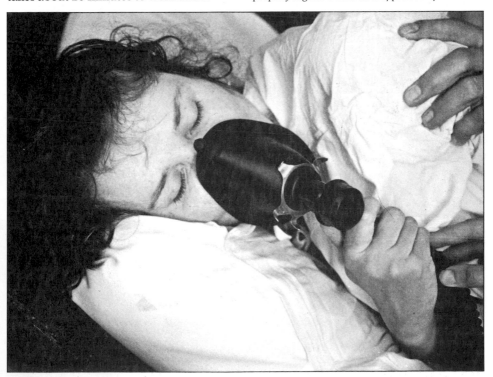

Anesthetics

These act by dulling your conscious appreciation of pain. A general anesthetic is never used during a normal birth; local or regional anesthetics can be given by injecting an anesthetic into a nerve root and numbing the parts of the body that it supplies. Local anesthetics are used before an episiotomy (see p. 186) and during stitching of the perineum after the birth (perineal infiltration) and if you need a mid-forceps delivery and you haven't had an epidural. This is called a pudendal block and is injected into the vaginal wall with a special needle that cannot injure the baby's head.

Epidural anesthesia

This has been called the cadillac of anesthetics and most people think it is the safest with the least side effects. It probably has no effect on the fetus directly but it does affect you in labor. One of the reasons why epidural anesthesia has become so popular in recent years is that it fulfills all the criteria of a good pain reliever but in no way interferes with your awareness and your levels of consciousness. There are very few side effects associated with the majority of epidural anesthetics, and for many women it is a perfect answer to how they want their labor managed.

HAVING AN EPIDURAL

An epidural takes about 10 to 20 minutes for a skilled anesthesiologist to set up. The effect is usually felt in a few minutes and lasts for about two hours but you can have more anesthetic when the pain returns and becomes severe.

Setting up the epidural
You will be asked to lie on your left side, pulling your legs up to make as tight a ball as possible. Your lower back will be washed with an antibiotic solution and then you will be given an injection of local anesthetic. A small hole will be made in your back with a solid needle and a hollow needle is then inserted in its place. Once the epidural space is located a fine catheter is threaded through the hollow needle and into the epidural space leaving a length of catheter protruding from your back. The catheter is secured to your skin along its length with paper tape. The local anesthetic is then given by syringe down the catheter and the opening is sealed. You will have a drip set up so that fluids can be fed to you intravenously should your blood pressure fall.

The position for setting up the epidural

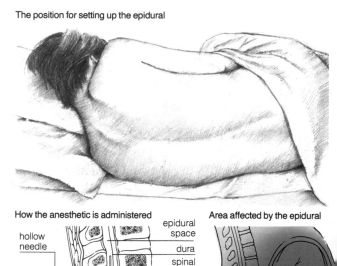

How the anesthetic is administered

hollow needle

epidural space

dura

spinal cord

vertebrae

catheter

syringe

Area affected by the epidural

Hypnosis

There's no doubt that hypnosis can afford relief from pain in a susceptible person. However, many practice sessions during pregnancy would be advisable and both you and the hypnotist (see p. 230) should be completely familiar with what is required of you.

Acupuncture

I would recommend using acupuncture for pain relief in labor only if you have found it successful in the past. For some women it will undoubtedly work but the acupuncturist (see p. 230) must be practiced at giving pain relief in labor.

Tens

This is transcutaneous nerve stimulation and advocates claim that it is a means of relieving pain in labor by stimulating production of the body's natural painkillers – endorphins – and by blocking pain sensation with an electric current. The electrodes are placed on the woman's body and she is able to regulate the intensity of the current herself. TENS has been used successfully in Sweden but it does not help everyone, particularly those women who experience a lot of pain in labor. TENS doesn't relieve 100 per cent of the pain but what remains is possibly easier to bear.

ADVANTAGES

1 It provides complete pain relief without dulling any of your mental faculties.
2 It has a tendency to slow down labor which can be useful.
3 No other local anesthetic will be necessary should you need forceps, vacuum extraction or episiotomy.
4 It allows you to be an active participant in your birth if you have a Cesarean section.
5 As it lowers blood pressure it is ideal for women with toxemia or high blood pressure.
6 The anesthetic can be readministered when necessary or allowed to wear off near the delivery so that you can control the actual birth. The contrations at this stage may be a bit of a shock though if you haven't experienced anything up until then.
7 It reduces the amount of work done by the lungs in labor and so can benefit women with heart or lung disease.
8 It reduces muscular activity in the legs and therefore is of value to diabetic women whose insulin and glucose requirements are therefore easier to balance.

DISADVANTAGES

1 Makes for a medically managed birth from the start.
2 The lowering of blood pressure may make you feel dizzy and nauseous. This is more likely if you lie on your back so turn onto your side.
3 There is the slight possibility of a post-anesthetic headache which lasts a few hours after delivery.
4 There is an increased possibility of an episiotomy and a forceps delivery. Depending on the concentration of the anesthetic, there may be a loss of muscle power and of the sensation of the contractions. This results in a slower second stage because you will be entirely dependent on the instructions of the midwife as to when to push the baby out. The length of the second stage is the factor that determines the use of forceps.
5 If the mother's blood pressure drops, the amount of blood supplying the placenta is reduced and so the oxygen supply to the baby is lowered.
6 Some types of anesthetics can slow the baby's heart rate down and so reduce the amount of oxygen available to it.
7 Not all epidurals are effective.

PAIN RELIEF IN LABOR

Type of drug	Action	Effect on mother and baby
Tranquilizers (Sparine, Phenergan)	In small doses reduces anxiety in the early stages of labor. Controls nausea, and used to lower blood pressure.	Doses need to be large enough to have the effect of reducing the mother's anxiety without sedating the fetus. Too high a dose may reduce alertness in the mother. A narcotic will probably be needed for the pain in the later phase of the first stage of labor.
Sedatives (Nembutal, Amytal, Seconal, Valium)	In small doses reduces anxiety and induces drowsiness. Helps sleep in early stages of labor. Valium can cause memory lapses.	Reduces alertness in the mother and can cross the placenta within 1–5 minutes. Sedating effects on the baby may last up to a week after the birth.
Narcotics (Morphine, Demerol)	Sedates and relieves anxiety and possibly relieves pain in the first stage of labor.	Reduces consciousness and tends to make the labor longer. Crosses the placenta in 5 minutes and can depress respiration at birth. Sucking may be inefficient (see p. 203). Can produce nausea in the mother.
Inhalation analgesia (Entonox, Trilene)	Relieves pain, can cause drowsiness if allowed to accumulate (Trilene).	Depresses alertness but this returns once effects have worn off. Makes you lightheaded while breathing in the gas. No significant effect on the fetus.

MEDICAL INTERVENTION

During the last ten or fifteen years hospital childbirth has been revolutionized by the development of new procedures which have been adopted in many as routine practice. All offer advantages, a few carry risks, though small. None of them should be used unless there are good medical reasons. Most people believe that the sole justification for their employment cannot be the convenience of the staff or even of the mother.

Episiotomy

This is the incision made in the perineum between the vaginal opening and the anus to facilitate delivery of the baby. It is the commonest operation in the Western world. The cut is made with scissors under a local anesthetic just as the baby's head appears. If done too early before the perineum has thinned out, muscles, skin and blood vessels are damaged and the bleeding may be profuse. Also the tissues are crushed by the scissors as they are cut. This leads to bruising, swelling and slow healing and accounts for a great deal of the

pain and discomfort which follows episiotomy. There is also the possibility that the integrity of the pelvic floor can be damaged if the muscle fibers are not correctly aligned. If the vagina and

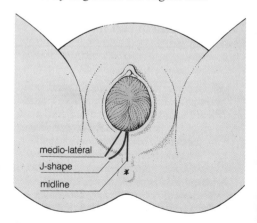

medio-lateral
J-shape
midline

Episiotomy incisions
These include the medio-lateral, from the back of the vagina out to the side; the midline, which runs between the vagina and the anus; and the J-shaped cut which combines the two.

perineum are stitched too tightly a woman may experience discomfort when intercourse is resumed. You might like to mention to your doctor that you wish to avoid being cut if at all possible.

There are grounds for suspecting that episiotomy has become obstetric fashion. If medical staff indicate that they think an episiotomy is necessary during labor, you should ask why it's being done.

Avoiding an episiotomy

You should make it known that you wish to find a good position for the second stage and that you'd like to avoid the lithotomy or recumbent position. A good semi-upright position will help to avoid the need for episiotomy (see p. 52). If your labor is proceeding normally, you should use this as an argument both for not lying flat on your back and for not having to have an episiotomy.

If you learn how to relax the muscles of the pelvic floor and allow your vaginal tissues and perineum to bulge out (see p. 113) you can avoid a tear. Familiarity with the sensation when the baby's head bulges or "crowns" will mean that you will realize that you are starting to tighten up in the second stage. You can try to do something about it.

Having an epidural anesthetic increases the possibility of having an episiotomy. If you do opt for an epidural, there is no reason why an episiotomy is automatically necessary but you will need to make your views known and try to have the end of the second stage well under your control by relaxing the pelvic floor muscle and not pushing down too hard when the head is delivered. I had an epidural twice but on neither occasion did I have an episiotomy.

REASONS FOR AN EPISIOTOMY
An episiotomy will be necessary if:
- the perineum hasn't had time to stretch slowly – breathing exercises and massage help with this
- the baby's head may be too large for the vaginal opening
- you aren't able to control your pushing so that you can stop when necessary and then push gradually and smoothly. An episiotomy will deliver the baby quickly if you have difficulty with co-ordination and control of pushing in the second stage
- the fetus is suffering distress
- you have a forceps delivery or vacuum extraction
- yours is a breech birth.

EXPERIENCE OF EPISIOTOMY
Sheila Kitzinger, in her study of 2000 women who had episiotomies, came to the following conclusions:
- They were more painful than a tear.
- The women found it more difficult to get into a comfortable position to hold the baby.
- The pain distracted them during breastfeeding.
- An episiotomy was more likely to give pain or discomfort during intercourse even three months after delivery.
- Two thirds of the women had never discussed episiotomy with medical staff during pregnancy. Some had tried but had been unsuccessful.
- About half the episiotomies had been done when the perineum was not sufficiently thinned out.
- More than half the women had not been instructed to release the vagina and pelvic floor muscles but had been encouraged to push instead making the cut more necessary.
- About one quarter of the women had not been told to stop pushing while the head was being born to give the vagina a chance to thin out.
- More than a third of the women were never given a reason for the episiotomy.
- Some women found the stitching painful but when they complained they were told that as there were no nerve endings there it shouldn't hurt.

Induction

This is the artificial "starting off" of labor should it fail to start on its own or your doctor decides that you need to deliver the baby early. The same techniques are used to accelerate labor if the contractions are weak and progress slow. Induction is planned in advance and you will be admitted to the hospital the night before you are to be induced. There are a number of ways this is done.

Prostaglandin suppositories

No-one knows exactly why labor starts but suppositories or a gel containing prostaglandins, which are made up of various hormones that have an effect on the pregnant uterus, are used to induce labor. They are usually inserted into the vagina during the evening and you should have gone into labor by the morning and not require any further intervention. This would seem to be the most satisfactory method of induction as you don't need any drips and you can therefore move around in the labor room.

Artificial rupture of the membranes

Also known as ARM or amniotomy, this is a method of stimulating contractions that is performed near to term as the risk of infection once the waters have broken necessitates delivery within 24 hours. It is not used as a method of induction on its own but is usually done during induction.

A pair of forceps or a tool not unlike a crochet hook is inserted into the womb and a small opening is made in the membrane so that the waters escape. For most women this is a painless procedure. Labor usually reaches full intensity quickly after ARM because the baby's head is no longer cushioned and presses hard against the cervix, encouraging the uterus to contract.

Amniotomy is now almost a routine during the preparation for any labor. If left alone, the waters don't usually break until late in the first stage. The two major disadvantages are that the labor becomes more intense and fast and if the baby has the cord around its neck, the loss of fluid increases pressure and can affect the flow of blood through the cord to the baby.

Amniotomy will also be performed if an electrode is to be attached to the baby's head to monitor its heartbeat (see p. 190) or if the baby's heart rate goes down, the amniotic fluid can be examined for traces of meconium, the first bowel movements of the baby. If these appear it can indicate distress in the fetus.

Oxytocin-induced labor

The natural hormone from the posterior pituitary gland in the brain, oxytocin, will stimulate labor. It is therefore used in a synthetic form to start labor off and keep it going.

Oxytocin is given in a drip. You could

Amniotomy
The bag of waters usually ruptures naturally towards the end of the first stage of labor. Before it breaks, it provides a cushion for the baby's head as it presses against the cervix (1). Once the membranes have ruptured (2), the contractions increase in intensity because the baby's head is now hard against the cervix. This speeds up labor which is why amniotomy is performed so often during the first stage.

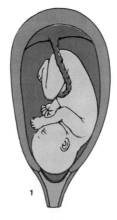
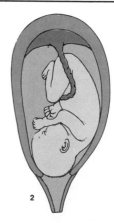

ask for it to be inserted in the arm you use least and check that you have a long tube connecting you to the drip. You should then have more room to move around, even if just on the bed. The drip can be turned down if you go into strong labor quickly and the cervix becomes half dilated. The needle won't be removed from your arm until after the baby is born. The uterus needs to keep contracting to prevent bleeding (see p. 178).

The contractions on an oxytocin drip are often stronger and longer and more painful, with shorter periods of relaxation between them. It depends very much on how your obstetrician handles the oxytocin. As the blood supply to the uterus is temporarily shut off during each strong contraction, it's thought that this may be detrimental to the fetus. Today obstetricians use oxytocin in as many as 40–50 per cent of deliveries.

One disadvantage of using oxytocin is that it may cause full labor to come on very quickly and consequently makes the need for a painkilling drug greater. Given that the rate of success with this form of induction is only about 85 per cent, its routine use cannot be justified.

Reasons for induction

Only 5 per cent of babies actually come on the due date and it's hard for some doctors and quite a lot of mothers to remain philosophical when that magic date passes. Both are concerned in case the baby is postmature or late. The fear is that the placenta may be becoming inadequate to support the baby and the baby is outgrowing its food supply.

Very few babies are truly overdue; 80 per cent of all babies who are born with a spontaneous labor without induction arrive after the due date. This is mainly because medical convention calculates the expected date of confinement from the last menstrual period rather than from the time of conception. Depending on the age of the mother, most doctors are equable about seven days latitude. After that, signs of postmaturity are carefully looked for.

Modern screening methods involve testing your urine for estriol. This hormone rises in the body throughout pregnancy and drops just before labor. If over a number of days your urine shows low levels of estriol, the placenta may not be functioning well. Obstetricians are very sensitive to the possibility of the placenta failing to function (this is known as placental insufficiency). Doctors might also listen to the fetal heart and check that it is satisfactory. If not, you will be induced.

However, waiting until the expected day of delivery is leaving it a bit late to face the prospect of an induced labor. This is something that should be read about and discussed earlier on in pregnancy. You and your doctor should try to agree on the course to be followed should induction be necessary in your case.

The older mother

Some doctors will state at the first antenatal visit that it is their intention to induce artificially an older mother on or around the expected date of confinement without waiting for spontaneous labor to begin. This is not always necessary. No doctor can ascertain during the first part of your pregnancy whether or not you will need to be induced. A mother who reaches her estimated date of delivery, given that she and the baby are perfectly normal, should be allowed to go into spontaneous labor. I would very much advocate, however, that she co-operates with the frequent monitoring of her condition and that of the baby once the EDC has been passed, and at the first signs of fetal distress, agrees to have the appropriate medical intervention.

ELECTRONIC FETAL MONITORING (EFM)

This is a method of recording the baby's heartbeat and your contractions during labor. It is the high-tech replacement for the ear trumpet or fetoscope. It is either in the form of belts strapped around your abdomen or an electrode rather like a tiny corkscrew clipped to the baby's head. The heartbeat and the contractions are recorded on a paper printout (see below right), which can be clearly seen by the staff. There may be flashing lights.

The internal monitor is the more accurate but the waters must be broken and the cervix at least 2–3 centimeters dilated. Two monitors are inserted; the

Many women find the monitors reassuring. They can see the contractions coming and prepare for them and watch their baby's heartbeat throughout the labor.

WHEN EFM IS NECESSARY

Monitoring the heartbeat and the uterine contractions is essential if you are being induced (see p. 188); your labor is being accelerated or you have an epidural as you will be less able to feel the onset of the contractions. Most hospitals now agree that EFM should be used routinely in high-risk pregnancies.

first is attached to the baby's head and picks up the fetal heartbeat, the second lies between the baby and the wall of the uterus to measure the pressure and rate of the uterine contractions. An external monitor can be used in early labor; one electrode is strapped around the mother's abdomen to listen to the fetal heartbeat and the other records

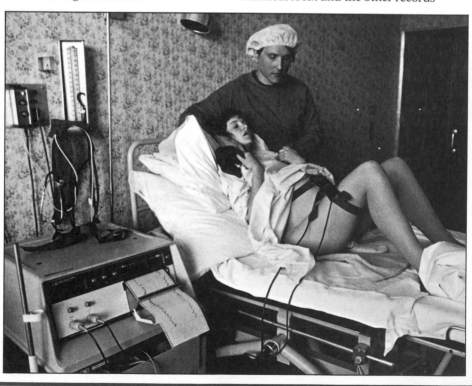

the intensity and frequency of the contractions. The mother is unable to move around during labor with these monitors in place.

In the United States almost 100 per cent of hospital births are electronically monitored and most hospitals feel very enthusiastic about EFM.

Advocates say that electronic fetal monitoring reduces the number of stillbirths and babies with mental retardation and brain damage during birth, claiming that in 10 per cent of all deliveries complications that cannot be anticipated beforehand do develop. Because EFM constantly monitors the fetal heartbeat electronically, it is said to be infallible where the human ear is acknowledged to be fallible.

DISADVANTAGES OF EFM
● The staff are more aware of any small changes and therefore are more likely to intervene.
● Three times as many babies who are electronically monitored are delivered by Cesarean section.
● EFM greatly increases the electronic paraphernalia in the delivery room and the atmosphere of the labor and birth.
● Staff are concentrating on the machine more than on the woman in labor.
● EFM restricts movement during labor.
● It may hurt the baby's head when the electrode is attached.

Telemetry

A method of monitoring by radio waves known as telemetry allows the mother to walk about remote from the monitoring equipment. The electrode is still attached to the baby's head but it is joined to a strap on the mother's thigh and not to a large machine. However, babies do suffer rashes where the electrode was clipped to them and there is no proof that they do not feel any pain.

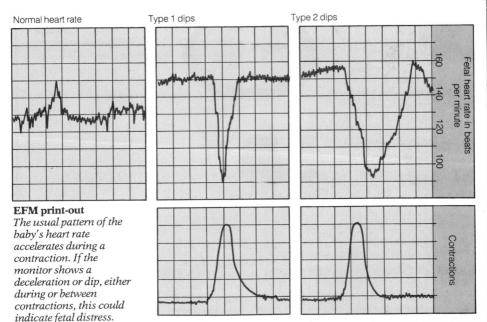

Normal heart rate   Type 1 dips   Type 2 dips

Fetal heart rate in beats per minute

Contractions

EFM print-out
The usual pattern of the baby's heart rate accelerates during a contraction. If the monitor shows a deceleration or dip, either during or between contractions, this could indicate fetal distress.

191

16 Complications of the birth

Even the best planned labors may not go according to plan. First labors particularly are so often not what was expected. You may have no idea what your threshold of pain is and become exhausted or your baby, through no fault of yours, may become distressed and need to be delivered quickly. You should think about the possibility of, say, an emergency Cesarean section or a forceps delivery so that, should they arise, you will know what to expect.

BREECH BIRTH

A breech baby is one that is born buttocks first. Most babies are in the breech position at some time until about the 32nd week of pregnancy, when they turn upside down (cephalic position) of their own accord. Four out of every hundred babies, however, stay put. If your baby is one of these, do not be concerned; most breech labors are smooth and the baby is quite normal though you will have to have the baby in the hospital. Your doctor may try to turn the baby during your prenatal visit by exerting gentle pressure on your abdomen. This is known as external cephalic version (ECV). It is a painless procedure but in many cases the baby turns back almost immediately. Don't try to do this yourself; the procedure requires the skill and experience of a doctor.

After the birth, your genital region might be slightly swollen but the swelling will subside within 48 hours. Breech babies may have bruises on the buttocks and genitals, but they will fade fast. You are more likely to have an episiotomy (see p. 186) with a breech birth. If you want to try to avoid one, and feel strongly about this, discuss this with your doctor during the first stage of labor.

The attitude towards breech birth differs on either side of the Atlantic. Most American obstetricians feel that a breech birth, particularly if it's the first baby, should go to a Cesarean section, whereas an obstetrician in Europe would not. In Europe, many mothers deliver breech babies vaginally and Cesarean section is justifiable in about one in six patients. Your doctor can be a determining fact in whether or not you have a Cesarean section for a breech baby.

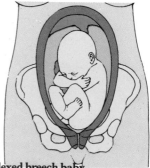

A well-flexed breech baby
The baby could be born vaginally, though an episiotomy will be necessary.

BIRTH OF A BREECH BABY

The baby's buttocks press against the cervix and effacement and dilation occur as with a cephalic presentation (see p. 164). The waters usually break early with a breech presentation and you will probably have bad backache (see p. 169) so kneeling on all fours will be a comfortable position during the first stage. For the birth you should prop yourself up in a sitting position though your doctor may prefer the lithotomy position (see p. 52) as you will need an episiotomy. Increasingly epidural anesthesia is being used for breech births. If you do have a Cesarean section, this will save time and allow you to hold and get to know your baby the moment after he is born.

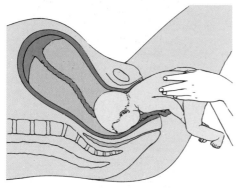

Delivering the body
The buttocks are delivered first and then the legs. While the body is being delivered, it is better to breathe through the contractions rather than to push. Before the head is delivered, you will have an episiotomy.

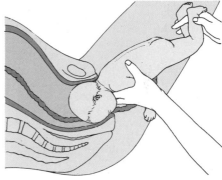

Delivering the head
The baby's weight draws the head down to the vagina and the body is then lifted to deliver the head. Doctors usually use forceps to protect the head and one push is usually enough to deliver the baby.

CESAREAN SECTION

This is a major abdominal operation and can never be undertaken lightly. There are slight risks associated with it such as the inevitable risk attached to having any general anesthetic and the risk of major surgery from bleeding or clot formation; there is also the disadvantage of being left with a scar on the uterus which may weaken it. Because the rate of Cesarean sections is rising rapidly there is some concern that the operation is being used too lightly.

You may know that you are to have your baby by Cesarean section weeks or perhaps only days in advance. This is known as a planned Cesarean section or elective section. Depending on the reason for the operation, you will either be admitted to the hospital for surgery or allowed to go into labor naturally and then undergo a "trial of labour" to see how you are coping. You may have a perfectly normal vaginal delivery. The Cesarean will be performed as planned before any serious problems arise. Unless your Cesarean is an emergency, it can be done under an epidural anesthetic (see p. 184) which is safer for you, and the baby and means that you can be conscious throughout and see your baby the moment she is born. Taking a part in the birth helps the vital bonding process (see p. 202).

193

Preparing for a Cesarean

Some women find a Cesarean section a great disappointment after looking forward to a vaginal delivery, especially if the hospital unit is not one that allows mothers and fathers to participate actively in the Cesarean labor and birth, and have immediate and intimate contact with the baby at birth and afterwards. Some women feel guilty that they've let their partner down and that he couldn't be there with them at the time of birth. Many mothers are angered and disappointed if they're not able to have their baby with them after the operation and have to be separated just at the time when mother and baby need each other for mutual support. But these psychological effects can be minimized if you prepare yourself for having a Cesarean section and look on it as a positive experience.

Ask to see your obstetrician so that you and your partner can have a relaxed discussion about what the operation entails, what the procedures will be in the operating room, whether you can be given epidural anesthesia and be awake and alert during the operation and whether your partner can be with you.

Through your own doctor or your prenatal clinic, ask if you can see a film of a Cesarean section so that you will know what is going to happen to you. You can also prepare yourself by talking to other women who have had Cesarean sections. This is one of the best ways of preventing you from having negative feelings about the prospect of a Cesarean birth. Not only will you get moral support but you'll also get useful information about how long it takes to be completely fit again after the operation, how to get in and out of bed, and how to hold the baby during the first days of breastfeeding. By talking to mothers who've had subsequent pregnancies after a Cesarean section, you can allay your fears about the future. A self-help group will be able to put you in touch with midwives and obstetricians who have a flexible and realistic attitude to pregnancy after Cesarean section.

WHAT HAPPENS

A Cesarean section usually takes about 45 minutes, but the baby is delivered within the first 5–10 minutes. The remaining time is for stitching the uterine wall and the abdomen.

Your pubic hair will be shaved, the epidural anesthesia will be set up, an intravenous drip inserted into your arm so that fluids can be fed directly into your bloodstream, and a catheter inserted into your bladder. A screen will probably be placed in front of your face and your partner might prefer to stand behind it at your head if he doesn't want to see the surgical procedure. The incision is usually horizontal and the amniotic fluid is then drained off by suction – you will hear this clearly. The baby is then gently lifted out either by hand or with forceps. You will then be given an injection of pitocin to make the uterus contract and stop the bleeding. You and your partner can hold the baby while the third stage is completed. If everything is all right you can start nursing her as soon as possible. Depending on the reasons for the operation, your baby may be taken away to special care for an observation period. The catheter and the drip will remain in for some hours and the stitches or clamps will be removed 5 days later.

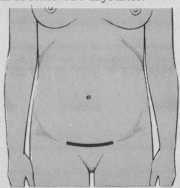

A horizontal line incision
This is common, for obvious cosmetic reasons and because the low, transverse cut heals more effectively.

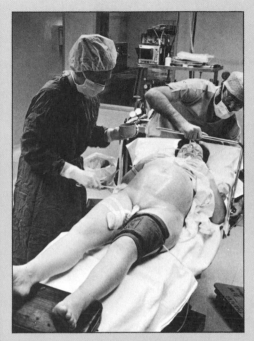

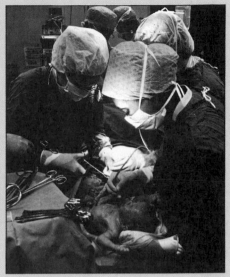

Once the epidural anesthetic is set up and you are prepared for surgery, the birth of the baby is very quick. Your partner can then hold the baby while your incision is stitched.

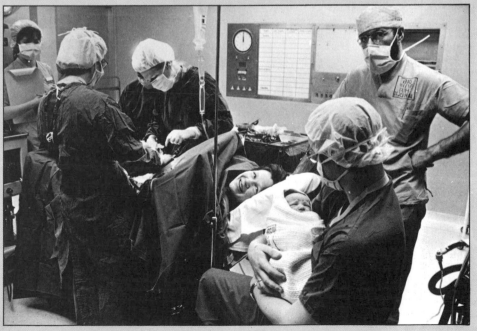

RETURNING TO NORMAL

After the operation you will be returned to the postnatal ward where you can be with your baby. Because you need plenty of rest in bed after abdominal surgery, you can concentrate on feeding the baby and getting to know her. You will be expected to get up and move around the next day and you can start gentle exercises (see p. 216) after two days. Most mothers feel physically normal from one week onwards after the operation.

You will lose blood from the vagina just as you would after a vaginal delivery. You must take care when lifting and refrain from strenuous activity for at least six weeks. The scar will fade, usually in three to six months.

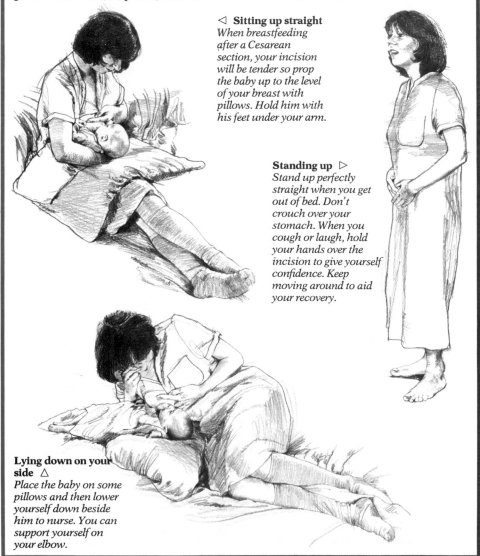

◁ **Sitting up straight**
When breastfeeding after a Cesarean section, your incision will be tender so prop the baby up to the level of your breast with pillows. Hold him with his feet under your arm.

Standing up ▷
Stand up perfectly straight when you get out of bed. Don't crouch over your stomach. When you cough or laugh, hold your hands over the incision to give yourself confidence. Keep moving around to aid your recovery.

Lying down on your side △
Place the baby on some pillows and then lower yourself down beside him to nurse. You can support yourself on your elbow.

REASONS FOR A CESAREAN SECTION

- Prolapse of the umbilical cord through the cervix
- placenta previa (see p. 144)
- detachment of the placenta from the uterine wall (placenta abruptio)
- fetus shows signs of profound distress; this will be obvious if the heart rate slows or "dips" at each contraction and, more seriously, between each contraction – this will show up on the printout from the electronic monitors (see p. 190); or if there is meconium in the amniotic fluid, the baby may have had a bowel movement which could indicate distress
- if the baby needs to be delivered early and induction and labor are considered to be an unnecessary risk to the baby or the mother
- if the fetus is extremely large or there may be cephalo-pelvic disproportion, where the baby's head is larger than the pelvic cavity
- breech babies are usually delivered this way
- a previous baby was born by this method; this is the commonest reason for the operation in the United States
- a uterine infection of any kind
- a serious infection of the vagina, such as genital herpes (see p. 60)
- the cervix fails to dilate
- forceps fail to deliver the baby
- serious RH blood disease

Some of the conditions that warrant abdominal delivery of the baby may not be apparent until labor has begun and this will then result in an emergency Cesarean section. You will be given a general anesthetic unless you have already had an epidural anesthetic.

FORCEPS DELIVERY

One of the arguments put forward by the advocates of natural childbirth is that forceps are being commonly required because mothers are routinely given drugs and anesthetics that interfere with their own efforts to deliver the baby. In other words, a certain proportion of forceps deliveries probably are doctor induced. For centuries obstetric forceps offered the only method of delivery that was not a natural one. As Cesarean section has become safer, the use of forceps has declined, so that they are no longer used for any hazardous type of delivery. Nowadays, forceps are applied only when the first stage is complete, the cervix is fully dilated and the baby's head has descended well into the mother's pelvis but has failed to descend any further, or there are signs of either fetal or maternal distress. The time to use forceps is a matter of judgment by your medical attendants, though most medical authorities consider that it's good practice to deliver premature babies by forceps so

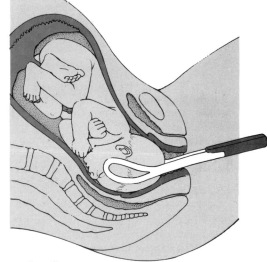

Modern forceps
These are designed so that they fit snugly over the baby's head. They are rather like a cage protecting the baby's head from any pressure in the birth canal.

that their heads are spared compression in the birth canal.

Your legs will be put into knee braces and a local anesthetic injected into the perineum. The forceps, which are shaped rather like serving tongs, are inserted into your vagina one side at a time and an episiotomy (see p. 186) is then performed. The doctor will have already determined where the baby's head lies, and with gentle pulling on the forceps for 30–40 seconds at a time, the baby's head gradually descends to the perineum. There should be no pain. When the head is delivered, the forceps are removed and the delivery is completed normally.

If longer forceps are needed to pull the baby out, you may be given a pudendal nerve block which is an anesthetic injected into the vaginal wall (see p. 184).

JAUNDICE

This is fairly common in newborn babies around about the third day of life. Medically it's called physiological jaundice, which means that it has no sinister connotations. A baby is born with a large number of red blood cells, which are rapidly broken down after it is born. When red blood cells break down and are replaced, they release large quantities of the pigment, known as bilirubin, which gives them their color and this has to be removed by the liver. At the time of birth a baby's liver is somewhat immature and is usually not able to carry the excess load of bilirubin, so the levels of pigments rise in the blood and give the skin a yellowish tinge. This kind of jaundice usually fades at the end of the first week when the liver has cleared the blood of pigment. The baby may also be rather sleepy. Jaundice can hardly be called a complication of birth, as it's really a variation of the normal.

To flush the excess bilirubin out of the baby's system, feed him often (wake him for feedings) and expose him to sunlight if possible. If the levels of bilirubin are high, the pediatrician may expose the baby to a light treatment (phototherapy). The baby's eyes are covered and he is placed naked in a crib under a light. The light breaks down the bilirubin so that it can be passed more quickly by the baby in urine. A more serious jaundice can occur due to RH blood incompatibility (see p. 150).

POSTPARTUM HEMORRHAGE

This is rare, largely because the uterus has a self-protecting device to stop it from bleeding. Once the fetus and the placenta have been expelled and the uterus is completely empty, it contracts down to about the size it was in the fifth month. The contraction of the uterine muscles squeezes the uterine arteries, nipping them so that they cannot bleed. Under normal circumstances therefore, little bleeding occurs after delivery and there is little chance of infection. (The lochia is a vaginal discharge and is only bright red for a couple of days – see p. 207.) A uterus that is not empty, however, is not able to contract down tightly enough to arrest bleeding from the uterine arteries and this bleeding is called postpartum hemorrhage. The commonest cause of postpartum bleeding is a small fragment of placenta left in the uterus, usually diagnosed by examining the placenta and finding that a portion is missing. Under these circumstances, the mother is informed of what is going on, is anesthetized and the placenta is gently scraped away from inside the uterus.

If bleeding occurs more than 24 hours after delivery, the lochia may become bright red again. This can occur even as a result of exercise, going shopping, carrying heavy weights or being too energetic about the household chores. Consult your doctor and you will probably be advised to rest for several days. If the bleeding recurs or becomes heavy, this can be the sign of infection or the retention of a small piece of placenta. Get in touch with your doctor immediately, Lie down and rest and feed the baby to release oxytocin to help the uterus to contract down. If you pass clots, call an ambulance and ask them to take you to the nearest casualty unit. Once you're in the hospital, you'll be given an anesthetic and the inner surface of your womb will be thoroughly cleansed.

PREMATURITY

This is not assessed solely on the time that a baby has been developing in the womb, but also on the weight that he has reached at the time he is born. The definition of a premature baby is one who is born before 37 completed weeks of pregnancy or whose weight at birth is below 5½lb. Small babies have a good chance of survival whenever they're born and a small but mature baby has a much better chance than a large premature baby. The cause of prematurity remains a mystery in about 40 per cent of cases, but various factors that predispose are pre-eclampsia (see p. 150), multiple pregnancy (see p. 147), premature rupture of the membranes and abnormal placenta. Some maternal diseases, such as anemia or malnutrition, and overwork can also have an effect. Fibroids and sometimes an ovarian cyst may be an underlying cause.

As a general rule, a premature labor begins without any warning and the first sign may be rupture of the membranes, the beginning of uterine contractions or some vaginal bleeding. Usually a premature labor is shorter and easier than a full-term labor, mainly because the head of the baby, the largest part, is smaller and softer than that of a full-term baby. Nearly all premature births therefore are

Parents can achieve a close bonding through the sight of their baby and touching him.

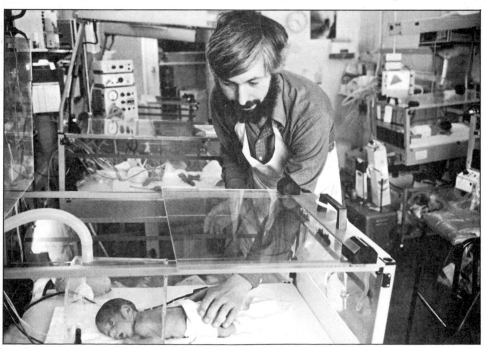

accompanied by an episiotomy in order to protect the baby's soft head from pressure changes inside the birth canal. Forceps (see p. 197) are especially useful with a premature baby because they're designed to prevent the baby's head from any damage.

The three most important aspects of a premature baby's health are his ability to breathe, feed and control his temperature. All these factors are taken into consideration if the baby is nursed in a sterile incubator where the temperature is controlled, where the oxygen supply can be easily changed according to the baby's needs, and where feeding can be achieved by a tube passed down the baby's nose, without pain or discomfort, into his stomach. Because so young a baby has a poor resistance to infection, the incubator is kept sterile and handling by staff and parents is kept to a minimum.

If you are afraid that the bonding that usually occurs immediately after birth may not take place with a premature baby, be reassured. The mother of a premature baby is encouraged to feed, touch and nurse her baby as soon as the baby's condition allows, but until that time she's encouraged to watch and join with the nurses in the baby's care.

Breast milk is particularly valuable for a premature baby. So if you use a pump your breast milk will be given to your baby and you can establish your milk supply so that it is ready for him when he can suck on his own. This is an effort that is worth making.

STILLBIRTH

A baby is stillborn very rarely – in fewer than one per hundred births. If the baby dies in the uterus before the 28th week, the uterus will go spontaneously into labor and a miscarriage will result. After 28 weeks the uterus will deliver the baby fairly quickly. Most women are aware that their baby has died, usually because it has not moved for 24 hours or more.

No one knows quite why a baby should die in late pregnancy, but in most cases it is thought to be due to an insufficiently healthy placenta. The placenta may have failed to grow adequately or become diseased in some way during pregnancy. Therefore it is unable to maintain an adequate oxygen and food supply to the baby. Occasionally the placenta begins to separate from the uterus and this can cause intrauterine death. Uncontrolled Rhesus disease (see p. 150) or poorly stabilized diabetes can also lead to a stillbirth. When the baby dies, most of the sensations of being pregnant fade quite quickly as the levels of estrogen and progesterone plummet. Even the uterus may diminish in size due to the absorption of the amniotic fluid from around the fetus. This may show up in the mother as dramatic weight loss which is why loss of weight is always taken seriously at a prenatal check.

If a baby's death is suspected, an ultrasonic scan will be done to try to detect the fetal heart. If the heart cannot be detected by the scan, it's unlikely that the baby is still alive. An X-ray examination can also confirm that the baby is dead. A baby's death can cause clotting problems in the mother and this possibility should be watched for.

The emotional and psychological effects on the mother can be extremely traumatic. A woman will quite naturally feel all kinds of guilt, inadequacy, self-loathing, sadness and depression and she may feel that she wants to withdraw and be completely by herself to come to terms with her grief. She may need the close comfort and support of an understanding partner, doctor or friend. Her needs must be sympathetically understood and met. Unless there is a good reason why a pregnancy should not be restarted, a woman who has suffered a stillbirth often finds that the key to normality and a return to happiness is through conceiving again, but all in good time. She should, once the sadness begins to subside, discuss this with her partner and her doctor.

Until recently it was always thought that labor should be allowed to start spontaneously – it usually begins within two or three days of the baby's death – and not be interfered with. Most women, however, find that they naturally want to have the dead baby removed as soon as they find out that it has died. In my opinion a woman's wishes should be paramount in this situation. With her partner she should decide what is to be done and if she wishes to avoid labor and have a Cesarean section, that operation should be made available to her. If, however, the woman opts to go into labor spontaneously, there should be no difference between this labor and a normal one. However, it is understandable that a woman's attitude towards her labor would be different and therefore she may experience more pain than she would normally when the labor has a happy conclusion. If labor is delayed beyond a couple of days, most doctors would advise that labor be induced with the best available method of pain relief.

Some parents who have experienced a stillbirth state that touching the baby helps to identify with the loss. The burial is also an occasion to help identify the object of grief. You can tell the hospital that you want to arrange the burial yourself if you feel this would help. Get in touch with others (see p. 229) who have suffered this disappointment – their experience can help you to understand your own reactions.

VACUUM EXTRACTION (VENTOUSE)

This can be used in preference to a forceps delivery, especially if the mother has already had an epidural anesthetic. It is used when there is a delay in the second stage of labor but where an easy delivery is anticipated. Unlike forceps, with ventouse the cervix need not be fully dilated. A small metal or plastic cup, which is connected to a vacuum apparatus, is passed into the vagina and applied to the baby's head. It takes about 15 minutes to get the cup in place. When a vacuum is created, the cup sticks to the baby's scalp, and by gentle pulling, and the mother pushing, the baby's head is brought down into the pelvis and then slowly and gradually delivered.

There are few serious complications with the ventouse. There is a slight swelling on the baby's head where the cup applied suction, although this usually settles down within a day or so of delivery. One of the concerns about a vacuum extractor, and to a certain extent forceps, is that they will be used to deliver a baby "expeditiously" as soon as anything untoward is noted, instead of allowing delivery to proceed normally, though more slowly. As the movement towards expeditious births gathers momentum, forceps or vacuum extractors are now used in about 65 per cent of hospital deliveries.

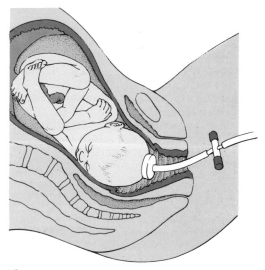

The vacuum extractor
Their use is largely confined to Europe; forceps are favored in the United States.

17 The first days

The birth of your baby is such a climax to the nine months of waiting that it can often overshadow the first few days. While you're waiting for your milk to come in on about the third day, you may feel excited or tentative or you may find yourself in a state of emotional shock. It's thrilling to explore your new baby and to enjoy quiet times together, but don't be surprised if at times it feels like a bit of a let-down.

If you are in the hospital for several days after the birth, it is important to learn from the nurses and experienced mothers in your ward. However, if you are a first-time mother, don't compare yourself with them and don't resent their experienced handling of their babies. The most important advice I can give you is to be easy on yourself. Don't set your standards too high. Don't try to be the perfect mother, and don't try to accomplish too much in these first days. Set reasonable goals for each day and take one day at a time.

BONDING

It's difficult to describe what bonding is; it's certainly getting to know your baby and exploring her through her senses and through yours – your eyes, nose, ears, fingertips and mouth, and even your tongue. It's also to do with attachment, protectiveness and possessiveness. This early attachment is possibly the strongest bond between human beings, and necessarily so, as it ensures the nurturing of infants, and hence the survival of the human race.

Establishing a relationship with your baby begins the second she is born. If possible you should be left in private with a minimum of interruption. Today a hospital birth makes this quiet peaceful time quite difficult to achieve. Babies do cry at birth but they usually soon stop and look about unblinkingly. If you are at home you will want to be in a low light with the baby nuzzled against your skin (see p. 49). If you are in the hospital you may have to ask the nurse to lower the lights and raise your hospital gown so that you can make skin contact with the baby. Don't feel that you have to take your baby immediately, you may need a few minutes to compose yourself. That's fine – let your partner hold the baby. Most mothers, however, do want to hold their baby immediately and no mother should be denied this right.

Research has shown that the sensitive period for bonding is the first hour of life. At this time babies are usually quiet but alert; they don't go to sleep for perhaps three to four hours. In this state they are responsive, and it's the right time for attachment to a nurturing, caring adult. It's also been shown that the first 30–45 minutes are the most rewarding for getting to know your baby through eye-to-eye and skin-to-skin contact. Try to see that you and your baby and the baby's father can be left alone for this period of time. Any cleaning up and stitching can wait. Looking into your baby's eyes renders her a person and not a thing; skin contact allows you to feel each other as warm human beings.

There's no question that all aspects of the bonding process – your voice, smell, touch, caresses, fondling – are good for the baby, but they're also good for you. The sooner you touch, hold and fondle your baby the more quickly your bleeding will cease, the more strongly your uterus will contract down and the better your breasts will respond with the let-down of colostrum (see p. 209) and later milk. You are also increasing your confidence in

handling the baby and helping her to adapt to a new environment. Studies have shown that a baby's adaptation is easier, smoother and more comfortable when it is held, soothed, crooned at and given the opportunity to feed at will. Soon after you take hold of your baby try putting her to your breast. Gently touch her cheek with your nipple and she will turn towards the breast instinctively. If she shows little perseverance – she may be sleepy if you had drugs for pain relief – express a little colostrum onto her lips to give her more incentive. Your partner can help by supporting the baby's head until you feel comfortable and natural.

The best time to build up a relationship with your baby is in the first hours of life. This is when the bonding instinct is most strong.

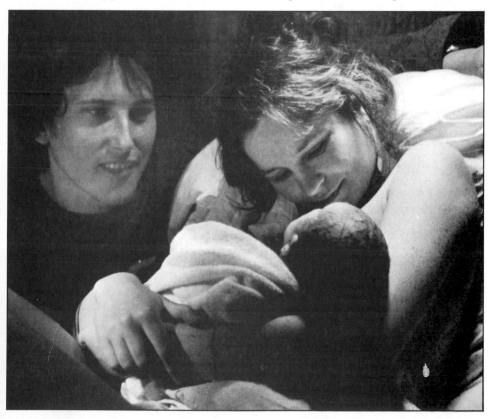

Importance of bonding

If it seems that I'm emphasizing this bonding process between parent and infant, I feel it's for good reason. Research has shown that parents who are given unrestricted contact with their children immediately after delivery raise their children in a more constructive way, are more sympathetic to problems, ask more questions, give reasons for their actions, and explain situations better than do parents whose babies are taken away at birth. A further part of this research has shown that at the age of five years the children who had had extended contact with their parents scored higher in intelligence tests than the control group. This does not mean that good bonding with your infant makes you a better parent or your baby a more intelligent child. What I think it points to is that it makes you a different kind of parent and possibly a better one.

FATHER'S FIRST CONTACT

It's probable that paternal bonding to an infant is not very different and certainly just as important as maternal bonding, so during the sensitive period it's important for you to hold your baby and make eye and skin contact. If you have been present at the birth and comforted your partner throughout the labor this is a good beginning. Be responsive to the cues that your infant will give you. It may take you a little longer and you may have to fit yourself into the role to achieve the same degree of responsiveness as the mother. All this can be helped by early and extended contact with your baby in its first weeks of life. Very often birth helps a man to express and enjoy emotions that society primes him to repress.

ESTABLISHING A ROUTINE

The first few days will be harder than you think; labor and birth are physically and emotionally draining. If you are in the hospital you are subject to the ward routine, which may begin as early as 5:00 a.m., and your day will be punctuated with nursing, changing and bathing the baby, mealtimes, medicine rounds, visits from the doctors, pediatricians, family, physiotherapists and friends. I had my first baby in the hospital and expected to have a restful time; instead, I hardly had a minute to myself, few minutes alone with my baby and was utterly exhausted at nights – I couldn't wait to get home and to peace and security.

Even if you have your baby at home you'll find that one job or activity succeeds another almost without respite, and that you will simply have to learn as you go. You may have read all the baby books that are available, but no book tells you about your baby. You have to take your lead from her as you try to learn her routine.

Babies don't know night from day and they require the same attentions during the night as they do during the day.

The smaller your baby, the more often you will have to feed her. Small babies, 7lb or under, require food at least every four hours and quite often there may be only three hours or two and a half hours between feedings. You should feed on demand; if you do, your baby will find her own routine faster than if you try to impose your routine on her. At least twice during the night your newborn baby will need a feeding and a diaper change. Nearly everyone I have spoken to seems to have had a well-behaved baby who slept for six hours during the night within a week of being delivered. Well mine didn't! The baby that gives you more than four hours' sleep during the night is an exception.

The best way to manage all that's demanded of you, to stay cheerful, and to get enough rest is to take your cue from the

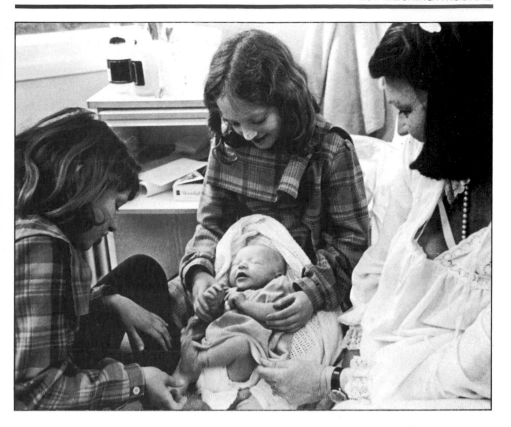

baby. You're going to have to learn to catnap because the only opportunity you may get to sleep during the first few days is when your baby is asleep. Just after delivery you have little stamina and will easily become exhausted from physical effort. Emotionally you are in a labile state because of the sudden withdrawal of pregnancy hormones. Little problems seem insurmountable and big ones insoluble. You may find yourself short-tempered and irritable with flashes of elation in between. You may be tearful and collapse in a heap as soon as anything goes wrong, and the next minute find yourself imbued with strong resolutions. Don't expect too much of yourself.

If you have a home birth, or an early discharge from the hospital, be easy on yourself. Don't worry about day-to-day domestic chores; let them pile up, as any

When you introduce your new baby to your other children let them feel and touch her too.

outside helper can see to those things. Save your energy to concentrate on what matters. There really are only a few things that should get top priority; the baby, then you, then your partner and any other children, then all of you as a family unit. Be unscrupulous in asking for help, even if it's only for the first week so that you have time on your own to get to know your baby and to work your day around her needs.

Most newborn babies have the same basic needs in the first few weeks of life, and once you have established a routine, you can then set about deciding what *your* needs are and how to best organize yourself on a typical day.

NEWBORN REFLEXES

Babies are born with certain reflexes which help them to survive the first days outside the womb. For example, babies put to the breast immediately after delivery will root for the nipple and suck to get at their mother's milk.

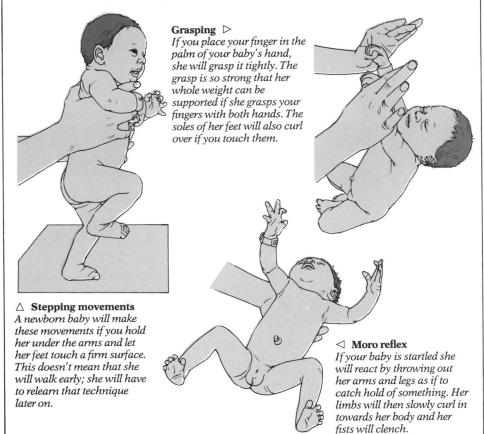

Grasping ▷
If you place your finger in the palm of your baby's hand, she will grasp it tightly. The grasp is so strong that her whole weight can be supported if she grasps your fingers with both hands. The soles of her feet will also curl over if you touch them.

△ **Stepping movements**
A newborn baby will make these movements if you hold her under the arms and let her feet touch a firm surface. This doesn't mean that she will walk early; she will have to relearn that technique later on.

◁ **Moro reflex**
If your baby is startled she will react by throwing out her arms and legs as if to catch hold of something. Her limbs will then slowly curl in towards her body and her fists will clench.

THE APGAR SCALE

When your baby is born five simple tests are carried out and marked to give an Apgar scale. This is an indication of her general well-being. The tests include:
- heart rate (above 100 beats per minute 2; below 1; absent 0.)
- breathing (regular 2; irregular 1; absent 0.)
- movements (active 2; some 1; limp 0.)
- skin color (pink 2; bluish extremities 1; blue 0.)
- reflex response (cries 2; whimpers 1; absent 0.)

Most babies score between 7 and 10. A second test is done shortly afterwards, about five minutes later, to confirm the findings and even if your baby had a low score the first time, it will usually have improved by then.

THE MOTHER

For the first seven days after the birth, whether you are at home or in the hospital, you should stay in bed for as much of the day as possible and sleep and rest whenever the baby sleeps. You will certainly be disappointed at your new shape. Your stomach will have sagged, your breasts will look large now that your bulge has gone and your thighs will seem heavy. Starting on your postnatal exercises (see p.216) will make you feel better.

Afterpains

Throughout our fertile lives the uterus never stops contracting; these contractions are felt as menstrual cramps at the time of our periods, as Braxton Hicks contractions throughout pregnancy and after delivery as afterpains. Uterine contractions after delivery are stronger and more painful than usual because they are the means by which the uterus contracts down to its former non-pregnant size. The faster and harder it contracts down the less likelihood there is of any postpartum hemorrhage (see p. 198). The contractions are usually not severe with the first baby but subsequently women become more conscious of them. They are also more severe in breastfeeding women. An excellent sign that you are getting back to normal quickly, they usually disappear after three or four days.

Lochia

For up to six weeks you may pass lochia, which is a discharge of blood and mucus from the uterus. Immediately after delivery it is like a pink or red menstrual flow; after a few days it becomes a dark brown, gradually fades to a creamy color, and finally becomes white. You should use sanitary pads as protection (super absorbent ones for the first two days) and delay the use of tampons until after the second week postpartum. Both the contracting down of the uterus and the cessation of bleeding occur more rapidly if you breastfeed the baby.

Bowels and bladder

You should get out of bed to use the toilet as soon as you possibly can after delivery and certainly the first time that you feel you want to. Quite often the bowels have been well cleared out at some point before or during labor and you may not want to pass a bowel motion for 24 hours or more. Don't worry about this but obey the first call to move your bowels and take care not to strain. Drinking plenty of water and getting up and walking about will help to get your bowels working.

There may be some hesitancy before the urine starts to flow. This is nothing to worry about and is usually the result of swelling of the perineum and the tissues that surround the bladder and the urethral opening. A good way to get started is to sit in some warm water, try out the Kegel exercises (see p. 113) and pass urine into the water. This is not unhygienic if you wash yourself thoroughly afterwards. You can also stand over a bedpan and if you've had stitches, this might prevent contamination of the wound with urine. Urine is sterile but acid and makes the raw skin sting. You might try pouring warm water over yourself as you are passing urine to reduce stinging.

You may also notice an increase in the amount of urine passed for the first few days. This is the way your body eliminates the excess fluid you have accumulated during your pregnancy.

COPING WITH STITCHES
Most stitches dissolve after two weeks. If you are bruised or the stitches cause you discomfort:
- sit on an inflatable rubber ring
- after bathing, dry the area thoroughly with a hair drier
- put salt in the bath to prevent infection and aid healing
- hold a clean pad against the stitches when you move your bowels
- don't get constipated (see p. 136).

FEEDING

Whichever method of feeding you have chosen, remember the colostrum in your breasts during the first three days is full of valuable antibodies which will protect your baby against all kinds of diseases.

Breastfeeding

If you feel that breastfeeding comes naturally, you may be surprised by how awkward the first several days seem. But don't worry. Establishing breastfeeding is always easier if you put the baby to the breast within a few minutes of delivery (see p. 203). Once you've achieved successful suckling in the happy relaxed atmosphere that surrounds the birth, you'll feel confident about future nursing. If this isn't possible, start nursing as soon as you can and try to relax and enjoy the experience. If you feel sore around the nipples, or your baby has difficulty nursing at first, remember that this is

Successful breastfeeding is always easier if you put your baby to the breast as soon as possible after delivery.

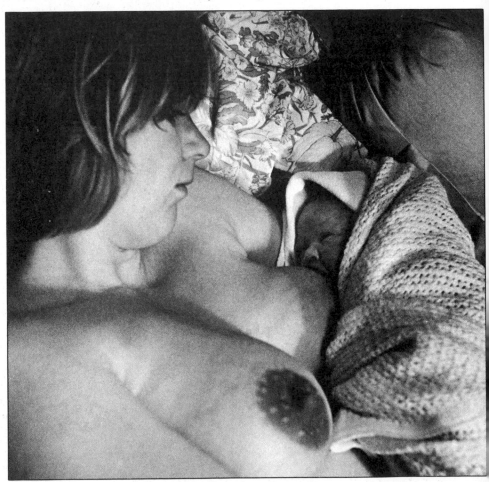

quite normal. Keep in mind that every woman is equipped to nurse her baby; no breast is so small it will leave a baby hungry.

Colostrum

During the first three days the breasts produce light, yellow-colored colostrum. It is a perfect food for the first days of your baby's life, containing water, protein and minerals in just the right proportion to take care of all your baby's nutritional needs. Colostrum also contains valuable antibodies which protect your baby against diseases to which you have developed a resistance such as polio and influenza. Besides all that, it contains a laxative which gets your newborn baby's bowels in motion. After about 72 hours, colostrum is replaced by breast milk, and for about two to three days, your breasts will feel heavy and full.

Let-down reflex

This is the automatic reaction by which the body makes milk available in the breasts. The reflex is a complicated chemical chain reaction of which you are quite unaware until you feel tingling in your breasts and then the milk surges into the nipple area. It occurs in seconds and is set off either upon stimulation of your nipple by the baby, your baby's hunger cry or even the thought of your baby. At this trigger the pituitary gland releases a hormone, oxytocin, which causes the milk-producing cells to empty their milk into the reservoirs in the nipple area. If you are not ready to nurse, press the sides of your breasts firmly to control the flow.

Getting breastfeeding started

In the first days the nipples are delicate and need time to toughen up so increase the length of time on each breast gradually. Two minutes on each breast will give your baby sufficient colostrum at first. Every time she cries you can try putting her to the breast, not just for food but also to get used to it. Make sure she is properly latched on (see below). Build up the time on each breast to 10 minutes each side by the time the milk has come in on about the third or fourth day. All babies suck most strongly in the first five minutes, during which time they take about 80 per cent of the milk. You'll soon discover when your baby is satisfied because she loses interest in nursing, she may start to play with your breast, or she may turn away and fall asleep. You'll know if she hasn't had enough because she will wake hungry and cry. At the next feeding, alternate the breast you start on.

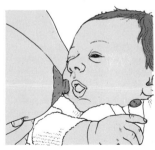

Rooting reflex
If you touch the baby's cheek with your nipple or finger, she will turn towards the breast and try to latch on. This is instinctive and can be further encouraged if you express colostrum onto the baby's lips.

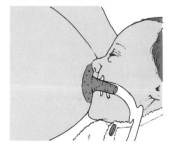

Latching on
The baby is properly latched on when the whole of the nipple area is inside her mouth, with her tongue underneath the nipple. She presses the top of her mouth against the reservoirs (see p. 83).

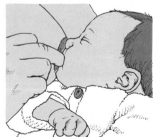

Breaking the suction
At the end of a feeding don't pull your breast away from the baby. This will make your nipple sore. Instead insert your finger into the corner of her mouth and gently ease her off the breast, or press down firmly on her chin.

Breast care

You will need to take good care of your breasts during the early days. Buy at least two of the best nursing bras that you can afford (see p. 125) and pay strict attention to daily hygiene of your breasts and nipples. Bathe them every day with water; don't use soap because it defats the skin and can encourage a crack or a sore to develop. Always handle your breasts with care. Never rub them dry; always pat dry.

After nursing, if possible, leave your nipples open to the air for a short time. Wear pads inside your bra to soak up any milk that may leak. Change these pads often; don't leave a wet pad in contact with your breast for any length of time. To avoid cracked nipples, apply a drop of oil or cream (arachis or olive oil or hypericum calendula cream) to the pad.

Tips on breastfeeding

☐ Give yourself time to prepare for nursing. Have a comfortable chair ready, and surround yourself with everything you need. If you're in bed, prop yourself up with pillows.
☐ Hold the baby high enough so that she can reach the nipple without effort. Cradle her head in the crook of your arm, support her back and bottom with your lower arm and hand. A pillow on your lap might help to raise the baby to your breast.
☐ Relax your shoulders. If you have to bend your back to lower the nipple to the baby, you will quickly become tired and your neck and shoulders will tense up.
☐ If your breasts become full of milk soon after a feeding, express a little (see p. 83) to help you to feel more comfortable.
☐ If your breasts are full and hard, the nipple will flatten out and the baby will have difficulty latching on. Express a little milk to soften the areola; as the milk flows the baby will latch on and suck.
☐ If you get too tired, you can express some milk and put it in a bottle for your partner or a friend to give to the baby.
☐ To ease engorgement, apply hot or cold cloths to your breasts. With gentle massage the milk with flow.
☐ If you develop a crack, express from the sore breast until the skin heals. Give the baby the expressed milk from a spoon if you don't want to bother with bottles and sterilization.
☐ If the baby refuses the breast it may be because she is having difficulty in breathing. Press down on the top of your breast gently with a finger to clear a space for her nostrils.
☐ If you feel feverish and notice a shiny, red patch on your breast, consult your doctor. This could be a blocked duct.

Bottle feeding

If you have decided to bottle feed your baby, you will experience about two uncomfortable days while the milk dries up in your breasts. You will be advised to wear a good, firm bra and to take mild analgesics if necessary to relieve the pain of engorgement. By the fifth day after your baby's birth, your breasts should be back to normal.

One of the advantages of bottle feeding is that the new father can be involved right from the beginning with feeding and feeding-time activities. It's a good idea for your partner to feed the baby for the first time within 24 hours so that he takes the plunge and gains confidence.

When you feed your baby, make sure

BURPING AND SPITTING UP
Some babies swallow enough air during feeding to cause them discomfort. Their piercing screams after a feeding are silenced as soon as the gas is passed. Other babies are never bothered by gas. If you aren't sure, hold your baby in an upright position and pat her back. If nothing happens, and the baby is happy, there is no need to wait for a burp.

Some babies spit up, others don't. The commonest cause is overfeeding. There is nothing to worry about, even if it looks like a lot. Have a muslin diaper ready or put a bib on the baby to catch the spit-up.

---

your back is supported and hold the bottle firmly. The nipple should be well back in the baby's mouth and should always be full of milk. If not, the baby will suck in air with her milk. If she shows no interest, encourage her to "root" (see p. 209) for the bottle by gently touching her cheek with your finger or the nipple. If the nipple suddenly goes flat, release the vacuum by gently pulling on the bottle. Allow the milk to flow again. Sometimes the nipple becomes blocked; change it for a new, sterile one.

Cradle your baby in your arms when you bottle feed, holding her close to your body.

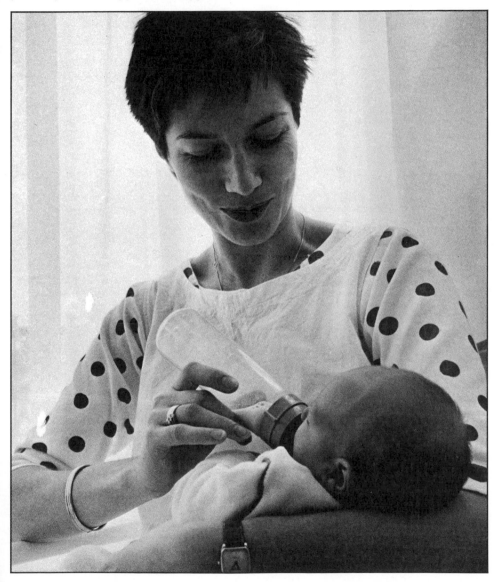

BATHING AND CHANGING

Until your baby is about six weeks old, the only parts that need daily bathing are the head, hands and bottom. To do this you need to "top and tail." Try to make it approximately the same time every day so that you can both establish a routine. Choose a time when she's awake but not hungry and irritable.

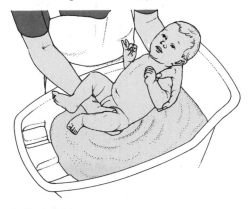

In the tub
Support your baby's head with your forearm and her bottom with your other hand. Her head should be slightly upright enabling her to look around. You can even start water games.

TIPS FOR BATHTIME
● Warm the room to at least 68°F and use water that is about 90°F so that it is warm and not hot when you dip your elbow into it.
● Squeeze a drop of liquid baby soap into the tub if you want suds. Even the mildest soap is defatting and dries the skin.
● Make sure that all the baby's things are ready and to hand before you start. When your hands are full with the baby you won't be able to reach otherwise.
● Wear a waterproof apron with a towel tied around your waist so that you can slip the wet baby straight onto your knee.

TOPPING AND TAILING

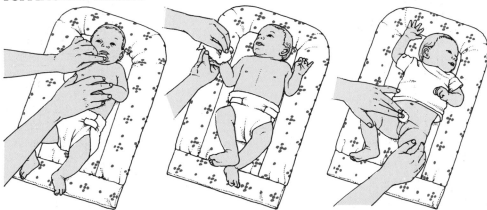

1. *Fill a bowl with warm water and place cotton balls beside it. Undress the baby, except for her diaper, and wipe each eye with a separate cotton ball dipped in the water and squeezed dry. Wipe from the inside of the eye outwards.*

2. *With another cotton ball, wipe around the creases of her neck, behind her ears, her face, and mouth and nostrils. Don't clean inside her ears. Pat the skin dry with a soft towel and wipe her hands and arms with a damp washcloth.*

3. *Put on a clean undershirt and remove her diaper. With a new cotton ball, wipe around the genital area, especially between the creases. Dry thoroughly. Most babies enjoy the freedom of not having a diaper on for a time.*

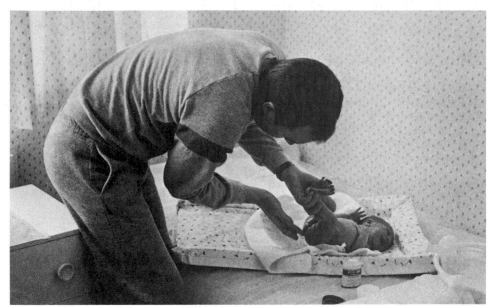

△ Diaper changing can be done with a minimum of fuss if you have all the creams and wipes to hand.

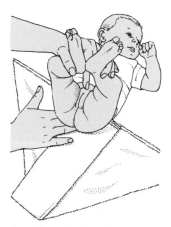

4. Rub on vaseline or ointment liberally to prevent diaper rash. Apply talcum powder on her chest and back if you want to, but not around the genital area, as it cakes when the diaper gets wet. Put on a clean diaper and clothes.

TRIPLE ABSORBENT FOLD

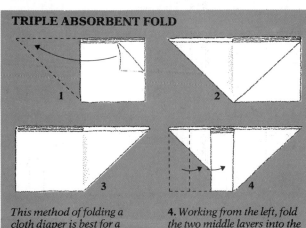

This method of folding a cloth diaper is best for a newborn baby because it has a thick absorbent central panel and it is neat when on.
1. Fold a diaper in four with the selvedges to the top and right. Pick up the top right-hand corner
2. Put out to form an inverted triangle.
3. Turn the whole diaper over so that the pointed edge is to the top right-hand corner.

4. Working from the left, fold the two middle layers into the center by one third and then fold in again by another third to form a thick and absorbent central panel. The central panel goes up between the baby's legs and the two points come in to meet in the middle over the central panel. Secure them there with a diaper pin. Use two pins on either side for a larger baby.

POSTPARTUM BLUES

A feeling of weepiness and depression is common around the third or fourth day when the milk starts to flow. If you find that your depression is more than just feeling a bit low and it lasts longer than two weeks, you should seek medical help immediately. Don't allow the depression to drag on because you think that it will disappear; early medical help may defuse the situation. Going without help may make your depression worse and mean that it will take longer before you begin to feel better.

Like any other depression, postpartum depression is more likely the wider the disparity between expectations and reality. Any negative feelings you may have, whether about yourself or the baby or about motherhood, will be exaggerated in the early days because of the fragile emotional state you find yourself in. This is no fault of your own, but due to your hormones which, after having been at very high levels for nine months, are suddenly plunged back to the comparatively low levels of normality. This enormous swing renders most women tearful, weepy, irritable, indecisive, moody, uncommunicative, anxious, insomniac and depressed. After the initial euphoria has worn off, reality seems difficult to cope with. You'd be absolutely wrong to think that the early days are easy. They are not. You'd be wrong to think that you have a lead on every woman and know how to manage the early days. No one does. The expertise, the tricks, the responsibilities of motherhood are acquired only through learning, which takes time. So be easy on yourself. Gather as much information as you can, read books, talk to the doctor, to friends who have had babies and to experienced mothers. Relieve yourself of unimportant tasks.

Don't try to keep up appearances. Let everybody but the baby fend for themselves. Be as open as your personality allows you to be. Consult your partner and friends about worries and problems. One of the best ways to keep the stresses, strains and new responsibilities of motherhood in perspective and prevent them from escalating into a serious emotional disturbance is to talk.

Rest and sleep

Sufficient rest and sleep in the first few days is essential though difficult to achieve. Many women feel totally exhausted after childbirth; it seems that your body is letting you down because it simply cannot function the way it did before you were pregnant. One of the reasons why you feel so exhausted is that the volume of your blood has been suddenly cut by 30 per cent. Therefore a volume of blood sufficient for your muscles to work efficiently cannot reach them, and so they feel weak and tire easily. It will take you several weeks, if not months to adjust to this enormous change.

You may be tempted to try some light housework or to go on a shopping expedition. But even a trip to the local supermarket can leave you exhausted, while such chores as vacuuming can actually be dangerous because of your weakened muscles. Try to be easy on yourself and avoid even moderate activity.

GETTING ENOUGH REST
● Never ignore signs of tiredness. Stop whatever you are doing, if it isn't essential, and lie down with your feet raised slightly above your head.
● You don't have to go to sleep to conserve your strength; resting will give your heart, lungs and other vital organs time to recover.
● Whether you have a hospital or a home birth, have someone to help with the household chores and the baby so that you can rest during the day.
● Discourage visitors if you feel unable to cope. Put yourself and the baby first and ask to be left alone.

Mother-love

Everyone thinks that mother-love comes ready-made with breast milk. This is not so. Many women would admit that they feel very little in terms of deep love for their baby within the first 24 to 48 hours. Love has to grow and the bonding process takes time. There is nothing wrong with you if it takes several days or even a couple of weeks. Mother-love is not something that can be pre-arranged; feelings of caring, protectiveness and love for your new baby have to develop in their own time.

Coping with being in the hospital

It may appear that the maternity ward is being run for the convenience of nurses and doctors rather than for mothers and babies, and to a degree this is true. You may not take easily to quite a lot that happens in the hospital. Nurses can be bossy and may not give you enough time to yourself or with the baby. It may seem that ward routines are timed specifically to interrupt your naps. It is frustrating to find that you have to take a hot drink just when you have dropped off to sleep. The hospital diet is not exciting and you may find the food badly cooked or too bland for your taste. Just when you need some time to yourself to recover, it is visiting time and you find that visitors tire you out too.

On the other hand there is quite a lot to enjoy while you are in the hospital. You'll have company and can share your experiences, observations and worries with other mothers. A pleasant social life can develop between mothers with new babies. Sharing their learning experiences and working out plans together, you may form new friendships which will last well after your return home. The companionship and friendliness that exists between mothers in maternity wards could be an advantage for you. You will find some of the nurses and midwives are supportive too.

If ward life doesn't suit you, you can make your feelings known to the nursing staff. There are many nurses who take an enlightened and flexible view and will do their best to accommodate you. If this isn't possible, you will find that your unhappiness deepens. It would be sad if the first few days with your baby were marred by the frustrations of the hospital life, so it would probably be better for all concerned if you asked for a discharge from the hospital early. If you feel that you haven't the strength of mind to make a decision like this, consult your partner and ask him to make a firm decision. The probability is that he will advise you to come home.

LEAVING THE HOSPITAL

Hospital practice varies, but whether you leave the hospital after 12 hours or six days, some of the following procedures will apply to your discharge.

● A doctor will give you a physical examination to check your breasts and to see that your uterus is returning to its pre-pregnant size and that your stitches are healing. The lochia will also be inspected to see if you have passed any blood clots.

● You will be asked about your proposed means of contraception.

● If you weren't immune to rubella (see p. 24) during your pregnancy, ask to be immunized before you leave the hospital. The vaccination will not affect the baby if you are breastfeeding.

● The nurse will show you how to clean the baby's umbilical cord if it has not already dropped off.

● The baby will be checked by a pediatrician; if you have any worries, ask now. You will be advised to take the baby to a pediatrician in a few weeks.

● You will be or advised to see your doctor for a postnatal check-up in about four to six weeks.

POSTNATAL EXERCISES

You should exercise at least once a day as soon as you can manage after delivery. It is, however, better to exercise for a short time, say five minutes, several times a day. Lie on your stomach for the first few days too to help bring the uterus forward into its pre-pregnant position.

The first days

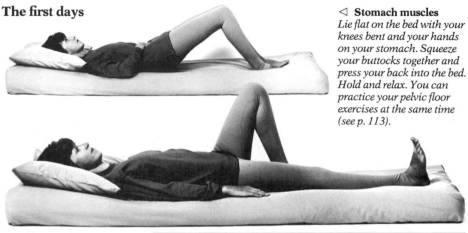

◁ **Stomach muscles**
Lie flat on the bed with your knees bent and your hands on your stomach. Squeeze your buttocks together and press your back into the bed. Hold and relax. You can practice your pelvic floor exercises at the same time (see p. 113).

△ **Hip hitching**
Lie on your back, bend one knee and flex the foot of the straight leg. Lengthen that straight leg by pushing your heel away from you. Then shorten it by bringing it up towards you (without bending your knee). Make sure you don't arch your back.

Foot pedalling
This is one of the first exercises you can do after delivery. This encourages good circulation and prevents your ankles and feet from swelling.

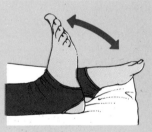

Basic routine

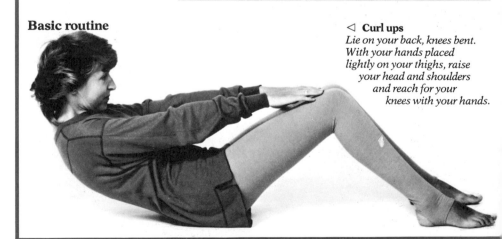

◁ **Curl ups**
Lie on your back, knees bent. With your hands placed lightly on your thighs, raise your head and shoulders and reach for your knees with your hands.

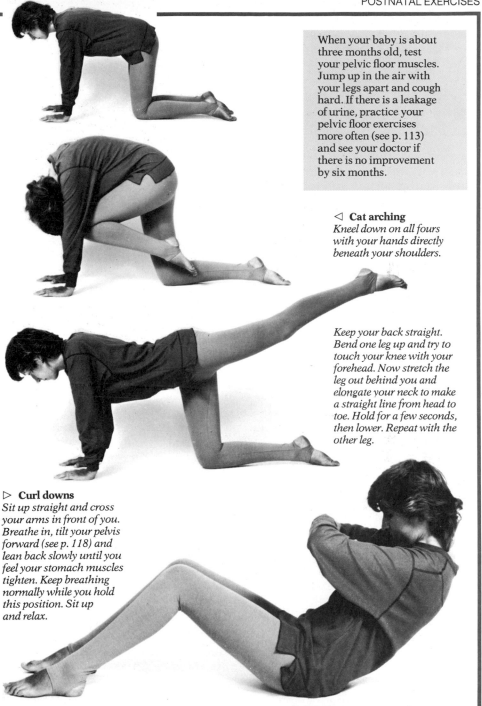

When your baby is about three months old, test your pelvic floor muscles. Jump up in the air with your legs apart and cough hard. If there is a leakage of urine, practice your pelvic floor exercises more often (see p. 113) and see your doctor if there is no improvement by six months.

◁ **Cat arching**
Kneel down on all fours with your hands directly beneath your shoulders.

Keep your back straight. Bend one leg up and try to touch your knee with your forehead. Now stretch the leg out behind you and elongate your neck to make a straight line from head to toe. Hold for a few seconds, then lower. Repeat with the other leg.

▷ **Curl downs**
Sit up straight and cross your arms in front of you. Breathe in, tilt your pelvis forward (see p. 118) and lean back slowly until you feel your stomach muscles tighten. Keep breathing normally while you hold this position. Sit up and relax.

18 Getting back to normal

Every woman feels differently after the birth of her baby. If the weather is warm and sunny, you may feel like getting up and sitting outside with the baby in the baby carriage beside you; if it is cold and wintry outside, the cosiness of your room will be what you seek. However, you should give yourself at least 7–10 days to build up enough strength before you get back to normal routines. If you had a hospital birth, and came home shortly afterwards, try to stay close to your bed until about the tenth day.

Coming home from the hospital can be exciting; you'll probably feel comforted and confident to be back amongst familiar surroundings. It can also be somewhat disorienting. In the hospital ward you had a routine organized for you, and everything was provided promptly. You weren't even expected to make your bed. At home you may be inundated with relatives and friends who come to see the baby. As time goes on, if you don't make plans to be mobile, to get out and about, you may feel shut off and isolated. The birth of your baby could open many doors to you. Previously your home may have been a resting place in a busy working and social life. Now you will be able to find out more about the community in which you live and what it has to offer.

THE NEW FAMILY

How much you and your baby will have established a routine largely depends on how long you opted to stay in the hospital. A stay of five, seven or ten days allows you to get to know each other and, taking the lead from your baby, you will have probably formed a loose timetable to suit his needs (see p. 204). On the other hand, if you decide to leave the hospital within the first day or two after delivery or had a home birth, your routines will be initiated at home and will be based on the day-to-day running of the household. There has to be give and take on both sides of course, but in most modern families the household does not revolve around the baby. The baby, though an important member, has to fit in with other family members and their affairs.

There's no question in my mind, however, that the quickest way to establish a routine is to let your baby lead you. You will want to organize yourself, your life and your interests into the time that he leaves you, after you have taken care of all his needs. It's easiest on the whole household if you wait and see how often the baby wants a feeding, how often he wants to sleep and when his usual waking times and sleeping times are, then try to dovetail your chores around his clock. One of the most important things for you to note is your baby's longest sleeping time. Try to fit in a nap during the same time.

Establishing a routine does not mean "training" your baby to eat, sleep and play according to a timetable that suits you. What it really means is feeding and playing with your baby when he's awake, trying to rest when he's asleep and fitting the rest of your life with him around this daily routine.

One of the early ways to introduce the baby to a diurnal rhythm is to make night feedings quiet and in a low light with as little disruption as possible. The daylight hours will then become synonymous with bustle and noise.

Sibling rivalry

If you have another child (or children) and are not having your baby at home, it is worth thinking carefully about how you are going to introduce your child to a new baby and so help to avoid jealousy. When you first greet your child, make sure that someone else is carrying the baby so that your arms are free to hold out, welcome him and gather him up for a cuddle. For the first few minutes give him all your attention, just as you would if you had been apart for any other reason.

Bring a present from the newborn baby – something that your child has really been looking forward to having. If he is physically capable, let him hold the newborn baby himself. Most young children are desperate to be of help, so encourage your child to give you all the assistance he can. During the first days and weeks set aside some times, several during the day if you can, which are just for you and him to be together, and which even the baby can't interrupt.

Don't break old habits just because the baby has come. If you had a special

Integrate your baby into family life so that he'll be entertained while you get on with other things.

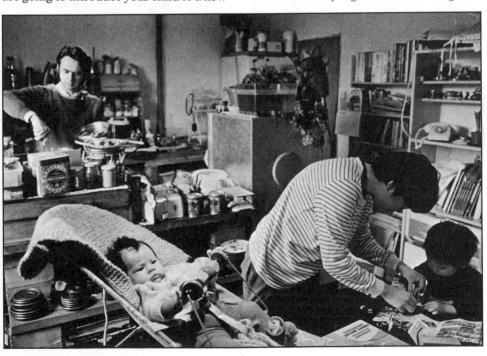

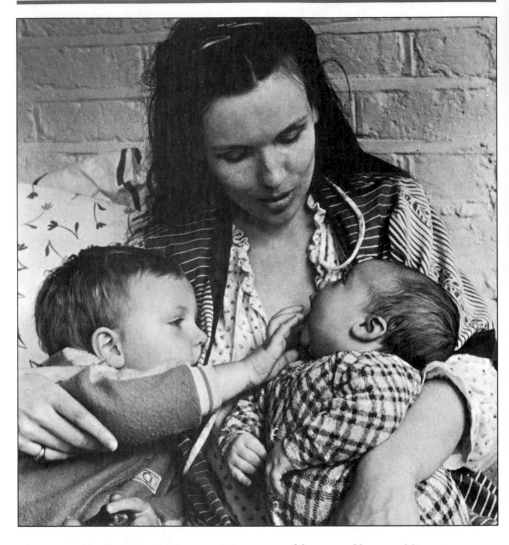

Closeness and involvement will help your toddler to accept his new brother without feeling shut out of your world.

routine at breakfast time or bed time, continue it with your child if you possibly can. Feed the baby just before these special times, so you won't be interrupted. When you have visitors, don't let them pay all their attention to the newborn baby; make sure that your child has at least as much. Praise and reward him as much as you possibly can and keep scolding to a minimum for a few weeks. If you are going to be in the hospital for several days, try to make arrangements so that your child can come to see you and the baby as soon as possible after delivery and regularly thereafter.

Your relationship with your partner

With a new baby, a mother starts out on an exciting relationship with another person and may feel little sense of loss

TIPS FOR COPING WITH TIREDNESS

Even if your baby sleeps well between feedings, your body needs to recover from the birth, and you *will* suffer from fatigue, particularly in the afternoon. To keep up your strength and good spirits and to get back to normal quickly, get as much rest as you can.

- Have a nap whenever the baby is sleeping; don't use this time for chores.
- If you aren't feeling well, don't be stoical; call your doctor. Your health could get worse.
- Continue to take your iron pills for at least six weeks after the birth.
- Keep to the balanced diet you had during pregnancy (see pp. 96–104) and pay particular attention to what you eat if you are breastfeeding. This is not a good time to diet. Your figure will return if you do your postnatal exercises (see p. 216).

- Drink lots of fluids; you will feel very thirsty if you are breastfeeding.
- Take meals and snacks that require a minimum of preparation such as salads, cheese, wholemeal bread sandwiches, fresh fruits and yogurt.
- Take all the short cuts you can think of.
- Use only disposable diapers at first.

- Take any offers of help for cooking and cleaning, so that you can relax and enjoy the baby.
- Let your older children help with the baby – tidying the crib or folding away the diapers.
- Keep the baby in the room with you for the first few weeks. You won't have to go far to pick him up and you can keep him in bed with you if you want to.
- Keep a couple of diapers in the kitchen, the car and the bathroom so you don't have to go back to the nursery at every diaper change.
- Believe in the fact that you need help.

when the closeness with her partner gradually diminishes. This is not so for a father, and a woman should remember this. A man's jealousy of his baby is not uncommon; many men confess to feeling pushed out by the baby and neglected by their partners. You must make sure that both of you understand that it is inevitable in the early days for the baby to become the main focus of attention. You will have to work to make time for each other. One way to resume your closeness is to take a nap together at the end of the working day.

One of the adjustments you both have to make is that no part of your life can be as spontaneous as it was before the baby. Even though you have to plan the moments rather carefully, you can have happy oases together in a day when most of the attention is given to the baby. But if you let your instincts have their way, your baby will probably always win, and you'll find that your partner gets less and less of your time and attention.

You'll also realize that you begin to feel differently about each other. This doesn't mean less, just different. It isn't a sign that your relationship is deteriorating; it is more likely to mature and become richer. Don't keep wishing that it was the same as before, because it never can be.

ADJUSTMENT TO FATHERHOOD

If you're relaxed and confident about the newborn baby, you will enjoy family life much more and your involvement will help you to appreciate that looking after a baby is every bit as exhausting as a day at the office or factory.

- Bathe and change the baby within the first few days and keep it up to give yourself confidence.
- Assert your right to have the baby to yourself for a time. Your partner will be glad of the break.
- Talk to your employers about the new addition to your family. If you have to get away early or adopt more flexible working hours in the first few months, they may be more amenable if they have had prior warning of your changed circumstances. You will also know where you stand in relation to paternity leave (see p. 228).

RESUMING SEXUAL RELATIONS

Your relationship with your partner changes in all sorts of way and for most people this includes sex. In the first few months after the birth, sex can be difficult enough to make you feel depressed about your new role. Some women lose their sex drive for a couple of months after childbirth and sometimes for longer. It's not uncommon for fathers to feel the same and temporarily to lose their ability to maintain an erection. Both of you must be prepared not to take this change of feeling personally. If you both can be philosophical and loving about your problems, you'll prevent them from developing into long-term obstacles.

When to resume sex

There is no magic date when you can start to have sexual relations again. To help you get back in shape, start your pelvic floor exercises (see p. 113) immediately after delivery, even though your genital area may be a bit sore. The ideal time to start making love again is when you and your partner want to, so discuss it and try it out tentatively. Take it slowly and gently. You may find that the tissues are a bit sore or tight. Glands that normally lubricate the vaginal area sometimes don't function for a short while after delivery so use a lubricating cream or jelly. It helps, too, if the vagina is well relaxed before penetration, so concentrate on foreplay before sexual intercourse. Try a different position from the woman lying on her back as the penis can press on the rear wall of the vagina, which may still be sensitive and slightly bruised. Your partner can help by gentle manual dilation if your vagina seems to be too tight. Don't be concerned about set-backs; they're normal. Try again gently.

Many couples resume sex comfortably at the time of the postnatal check-up. But if you've had an episiotomy you'll be sore and tender for longer, and your partner should not attempt penetration until you feel comfortable. However, this does not disbar gentle exploration. Also, while you are breastfeeding, your breasts may feel sore and heavy and if you have a cracked or sore nipple, fondling will be out of the question.

If after several months one of you is still feeling reluctant to resume your sexual relationship, do ask for help. You'll be surprised how much easier it is once you've talked to someone and it may be easier for you both to talk with a third party, perhaps a friend or a relative or a sex therapist. The most important thing is to talk about your feelings and keep channels of communication with your partner open.

LOSS OF LIBIDO

● Many women feel unattractive; your body will still be out of shape compared to your pre-pregnancy figure. It's difficult to feel sexually attractive if you have a poor self-image (see p. 90).

● The presence of the baby may be a stumbling block to expressions of love and sexual interest, especially if he is sleeping in the same room.

● You will both be feeling tired, which does tend to inhibit normal sexual urges.

● You may be suffering from physical blocks to satisfactory sex and so are loathe to try again.

● Parents do become very baby-oriented in the first few weeks, and you may feel that there isn't room for anyone else in your emotions. This is perfectly natural. What you should do is tell your partner about your feelings. You'll probably both feel this way to some degree.

● Many of the daily activities surrounding babies may make you feel unattractive – washing diapers, and smells of spit-up – all these things can be a bit off-putting.

CONTRACEPTION

Even though you are breastfeeding, or haven't restarted menstruating, you are unprotected and should use some form of contraceptive device when you resume intercourse. If you breastfeed your baby totally, your periods will probably not return until you wean him; if you don't breastfeed, or only for a short time, your periods should return sometime between two and four months after the birth. You will be asked before you are discharged from the hospital about your planned form of contraception and you may want to decide on something at this time rather than wait until your postnatal check-up, which is usually sometime between four and six weeks after the birth, to arrange it.

The pill
If you don't breastfeed, you can take the combined contraceptive pill. This is not a suitable method of contraception if you are breastfeeding, however. The combined pill contains estrogen, which interferes with your metabolism and could have an inhibiting effect on milk production.

During your pregnancy and after the birth you may have suffered certain conditions for the first time and you would therefore be unwise to use the contraceptive pill if you have
- *high blood pressure*
- *diabetes*
- *postnatal depression*

Cervical cap
You may have to be fitted for a new, larger cap if your old one is no longer reliable. Use it in conjunction with a spermicidal cream or jelly. You will not have a fitting for a cervical cap until your postnatal check-up, about six weeks after the birth. Check the size again around six to nine months in case you need another change in size. If you're happy with it, this method is ideal for the somewhat sporadic lovemaking of new parents.

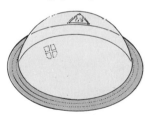

cervical cap

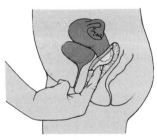

Checking position of cap
Before intercourse always check that the rubber dome of the cap covers the cervix completely.

Intra-uterine device (IUD)
An IUD will be inserted at your postnatal check-up. If you were worried about it before, the insertion of an IUD is much easier once you have had a baby.

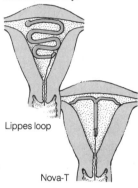

Lippes loop

Nova-T

Condom
This is the easiest method to use before your check-up. Use plenty of spermicidal jelly or cream with the condom as your vagina will be less well lubricated.

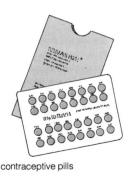

contraceptive pills

POSTNATAL CHECK-UP

This is usually done between four and six weeks after delivery. You will have an obstetric and medical check-up and at the same time you should ask questions about anything that is bothering you in order to sort out problems and gain reassurance. These questions can be about any subject, about the baby, your own well-being, sex, feeding, crying, routines – about anything that you feel needs clarifying.

During your medical check-up your blood pressure will be checked and your weight noted, your nipples and breasts will be examined, your abdomen will be palpated to check that the uterus has contracted down to its pre-pregnant size, and you'll have an internal examination and a smear test for cancer of the cervix. If you're suffering from any bladder discomfort or pain when you move your bowels, you should alert your doctor.

You should also discuss contraception (see p. 223). A perfect time to have an IUD or a cervical cap fitted is during the internal examination. The doctor will also check the scar if you had any stitching.

The baby's first check-up

Your pediatrician will want to see the baby within a few weeks of birth. At this first visit it is usual for the baby to be weighed and to have his eyes, cord, genitalia, and skin checked and for you to have a general discussion with the doctor about how feeding is going. This would be the time to raise any queries you might have about the daily care of the baby and what you might expect to happen over the next few weeks and months and to find out the timetable for immunization against the infectious childhood illnesses – diphtheria, tetanus, polio, whooping cough, measles and rubella. The polio vaccine is given by mouth. It is important that all children where possible should be immunized as this has proved to be a thoroughly successful form of preventative medicine.

GOING BACK TO WORK

Having committed yourself to this while you were pregnant (see p. 40), you may need to rethink it, depending on your circumstances. It is a good idea to include your doctor in this decision, as there are many factors affecting your health and that of the baby about which your doctor can advise you. You should start finding a good system of childcare about six weeks before you intend to return to work. You will need to begin weaning the baby from the breast then too, at least during the day.

If you do begin working before the baby is four months old, and therefore before any mixed feeding, you will need to plan. Introduce a routine so that feeding times are predictable and constant. Nurse the baby at breakfast and around 6 p.m.; the person who looks after him need give only the expressed milk or milk substitute for the other two daytime feedings. If you don't want your baby to take any milk

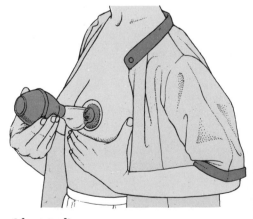

A breast reliever
This is particularly useful to keep at work. It is compact and can express a little milk quickly if you feel uncomfortable. It is helpful for drawing your nipple out so the baby can latch on.

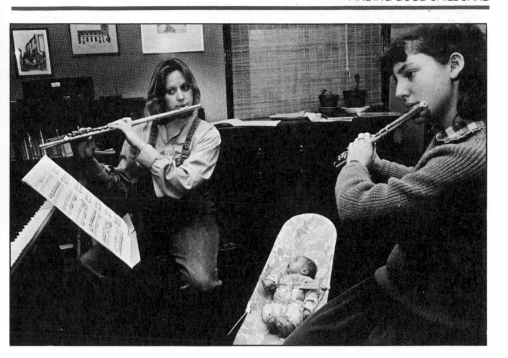

If you are lucky enough to have freelance work in your own home, the baby can join in too.

substitutes, start freezing expressed breast milk in advance; it will keep for several weeks in a freezer kept at 0°F. It should take around two weeks to get into this routine. Unless you plan to express milk at work, you will need to run down your daytime milk production or you will be most uncomfortable.

Finding good childcare

Governments tend not to give high priority to providing suitable childcare for parents of pre-school children. You will therefore need to ask around amongst your friends, neighbors, local government, churches and independent groups to find out what provision there is in your area.

You may be lucky enough to have a relative or friend who will look after the baby. Other options include:
☐ Full-time babysitter/housekeeper – while this is probably the most expensive option, it also may give you the peace of mind of knowing that your baby is well cared for in his own home by a competent "mother substitute." The right person is

hard to find, however; in addition to asking around, you might try calling childcare agencies and placing an advertisement in your local newspaper. Perhaps you could share a full-time babysitter with another family. If you want someone who lives in, you might consider an *au pair* as well.
☐ Family daycare – with this less expensive option you take your baby to the home of a woman who lives nearby and cares for several children at home – usually no more than four or five in addition to her own.
☐ Licensed daycare centers – good quality group daycare can be difficult to find. Check with your local government, YWCA and churches in your area. Private industry is also entering this field; check your yellow pages.
☐ On-site daycare – few companies offer daycare on the premises, but if yours does, be sure to reserve a place in advance.

ENJOYING PARENTHOOD

I have spoken to many mothers who felt that they had reached the end of their tether within the first few weeks of having a baby. It is important for you to release your pent-up feelings and ease tension and anxiety and enjoy being a parent.

□ You really don't have to bother about giving babycare a high priority; you automatically will. What you have to make an effort to do is to give care of yourself a higher priority than most reasonable women want to do. Try to be a little more selfish than you want to be by replacing the less important babycare activities with care of yourself. Your ultimate aim should be your own peace of mind and happiness; don't make the mistake of aiming for what other people would consider to be expert babycare. This is particularly important if you are breastfeeding; you must be fit and rested.

□ Even in the early days when you're drawn to be with your baby most of the time, it's essential to have some time on your own, so do whatever you have to do to get it. Perhaps you could arrange with a friend to leave your baby with her for an afternoon a week; you can do the same for her. You might like to make this a permanent arrangement.

□ Don't isolate yourself for too long. Often during the early weeks, you may feel agoraphobic and want to keep safe inside the house with your baby, away from traffic noise and the outside world. If this is your first child, start building up a circle of contacts, either through an independent group or making friends with other women in the hospital. You could join or set up a babysitting co-op in your area.

□ Find out about the play groups and community centers in your area and see what they have to offer. They may provide babysitting services while you attend a dance class or discussion group.

□ Don't expect too much of yourself and don't expect too much of your baby. You aren't perfect, but neither is your baby, and you have to forgive imperfections in him as well as yourself. Don't set impossibly high standards of mother or baby behavior. Be prepared to be as flexible as you possibly can in your care of the baby.

□ Most people find the first weeks with a baby scary. As a doctor I did with each of my children and longed for reassurance. What you can rest on is the sure knowledge that mothers have taken care of their infants instinctively for millennia, and *you* are endowed with the same abilities as those mothers.

CRYING

Babies sleep a lot during the first few months, but they also appear to cry a lot. If you feel that your baby never stops crying, make a written note of his feeding, sleeping and crying pattern over a 24-hour period. You may be surprised to find that your baby was awake for about 4 hours out of the 24.

Crying is the means by which your baby communicates with you. Check the following possible causes:

● Is he hungry? Even if he was fed only two hours ago, he just might want some more now.

● Check his diaper, it could be wet or dirty. Most babies don't seem to mind a wet diaper, but a few object strongly to a dirty one.

● Is his room warm enough? Babies need a constant temperature of about 70°F, even at night. If he is too hot, remove some of the covers. A number of light covers are more effective than one thick one.

● He may be bored and lonely and want company. If you are doing something else, an infant seat props him up and allows him to see what is going on, or you can put him in a sling and carry him about.

A contented new family member brings a happy ending to the months of planning and preparation.

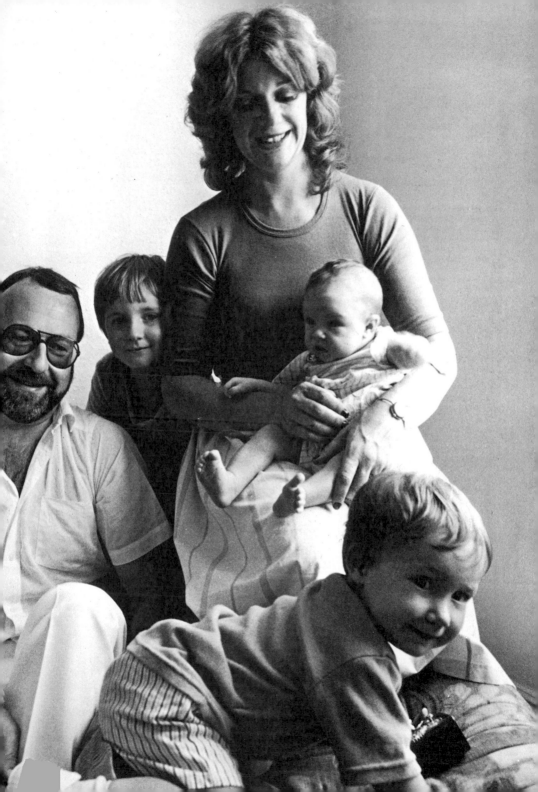

Appendix

Request for minimal intervention in hospital delivery

In order to make your feelings and preferences clear to the medical staff who attend you at your delivery you might like to write a letter to your doctor, clinic or the hospital.

Dear . . . . . .

I am writing to you to make clear my feelings about my forthcoming labor and delivery. I want to look on my labor as a normal event rather than a medical disorder. I would like to feel that it is possible to have my baby with no equipment or drugs unless my labor proves complicated and abnormal, in which case I would be very grateful for a discussion about the complications and the medical expertise and equipment in the hospital.

Throughout my pregnancy I will have good prenatal care and I will practice the psychoprophylactic technique in preparation for childbirth. The baby's father is also familiar with the technique and I want him (or my chosen birth assistant) to be by my side at all times throughout my labor.

I do not want and do not consent to any of the following:
- shaving of my pubic hair
- an enema, unless I have constipation
- a routine episiotomy
- any drugs given to me or my baby without adequate discussion and my express permission in each instance
- any mechanical fetal monitoring.

I also request the following:
- I would like to help deliver my baby onto my stomach.
- I would prefer that the cord is not cut until it has stopped pulsating, unless there is a specific reason.
- After delivery, providing all is well, I would like my baby to be left with me for as long as I want so that we may get to know him or her and I may start breastfeeding straight away.
- I would like to keep my baby with me during my stay in the hospital so that I can breastfeed on demand. I would be grateful for any help from the staff at any time. Should the baby need water in the first few days, I wish it to be plain boiled water from a spoon.

I do not wish to appear aggressive or antagonistic, but I think you will agree that it is a good idea to state my wishes clearly in writing so that there are no misunderstandings. I would appreciate confirmation in writing that this letter has been placed on file.

Sincerely yours,

Rights and benefits

The Pregnancy Discrimination Act of 1978 (PDA) requires employers to treat pregnancy-related illnesses on an equal basis with all other medical conditions. The principle is "equal coverage for pregnancy." If an employer offers disability benefits, sick leave and health insurance for other conditions, these benefits must also be applied to pregnancy. However, PDA applies only to firms with 15 employees or more, and only to benefits already in place. Although many women would argue that pregnancy is hardly a "sickness," if a company has no sick leave policy, it is not required to provide such a policy for the pregnant woman. Not surprisingly, policies and practices vary widely around the country.

Eligibility for disability coverage

You are eligible for disability coverage only as long as you are considered medically unable to work. Your employer may ask you to submit a doctor's statement certifying that you are incapable of returning to work. Alternatively, you may be asked to be examined by the company doctor.

Maternity leave

Employers can offer three types of leave policies, either singly or in combinaton.

● *Disability* – paid leave which applies to the mother during the time she is physically disabled as certified by a doctor.

● *Paid leave* – this type of leave is granted to mothers to allow them to spend some time with their baby without a complete loss of pay. The woman's job continues to be guaranteed to her upon her return.

● *Unpaid leave* – offers mothers additional time with the baby, again with a job guarantee upon her specified return. Check with your employer to find out what options you have.

Paternity leave

While there is no provision in law for paternity leave, an increasing number of companies offer some leave time to new fathers. However, few new fathers take more than two weeks of leave time – and often they use their accrued vacation time for this purpose.

Health insurance

Under PDA, health insurance must cover pregnancy and delivery in the same way as other medical conditions. Rates of payment, too, must be the same. But check your health insurance carefully; normally an employer does not have to provide coverage for you if you are pregnant when you begin a new job, for instance.

Useful addresses

International Childbirth Education Association (ICEA) P.O. Box 20048
P.O. Box 20048
Minneapolis, Minn. 55420
A nationwide organization dedicated to family-centered maternity care and freedom of choice in childbirth. Encourages you to write with questions concerning childbirth education, or related topics. Will refer you to the Childbirth Education Association in your area. Publishes periodicals, newsletters, books and other resource materials.

LaLeche League Internatonal
9616 Minneapolis Avenue
Franklin Park, Ill. 60131
A nationwide organization of women who have breastfed and can offer practical advice and support. Organizes local monthly meetings and supplies information through publications, meetings, telephone service and correspondence.

American Society for Psychoprophylaxis in Obstetrics (ASPO)/Lamaze
1840 Wilson Blvd.
Suite 204
Arlington, Va. 22201
A nationwide organization devoted to the Lamaze method of childbirth. Offers a referral service for certified Lamaze instructors in your area. Publishes a brochure on the Lamaze method, as well as Genesis, *a magazine on pregnancy, childbirth and early childhood.*

International Association of Parents and Professionals for Safe Alternatives in Childbirth (NAPSAC)
P.O. Box 428
Marble Mill
Miss. 63764
Promotes safe, family-centered childbirth. Of particular interest to women who want home birth. Publishes an alternative birth services directory listing doctors, midwives, and home birth attendants. Has a quarterly newsletter and mail-order bookstore.

Planned Parenthood Federation of America, Inc.
810 Seventh Avenue
New York, N.Y. 10019
Clinics in 45 states and the District of Columbia offer a

229

wide variety of reproductive health services including tests for pregnancy, prenatal care and infertility programs. Counselling and referral services are also available.

Maternity Center Association
48 E. 92nd St.
New York, N.Y. 10028
A national health agency offering a variety of services for families interested in alternatives to hospital birth.

U.S. Department of Health and Human Services
Office of Human Developmental Services
Washington, D.C. 20201
A federal agency providing a number of programs and services for children and families. The Administration for Children, Youth and Families publishes free or inexpensive material for parents. Write for a catalogue from Library and Statutory Distribution Service, Department 76, Washington, D.C. 20401

Family Focus
2300 Green Bay Road
Evanston, Ill. 60201
A private, nonprofit agency providing models for starting community-based support groups for expectant parents and families with young children. Offers information on forming self-help groups and family support centers.

MELD
123 East Grant Street
Minneapolis, Minn. 55403
Provides information and support to first-time parents, using a self-help group approach. Provides information on forming a support group for a two-year period from prenatal to two-years-old.

American Academy of Husband-Coached Childbirth
P.O. Box 5224
Sherman Oaks, Ca. 91413
Provides information on prepared childbirth involving the partner.

American College of Nurse Midwives
1522 K. St. N.W.
Washington, D.C. 20005
Provides information on midwife-assisted childbirth and prenatal care.

Day Care Council of America
1602 17th Street, N.W.
Washington, D.C. 20009
A clearinghouse for daycare-related information and resources.

Mother's Center
c/o Marge Milch/Lorraine Slepian
129 Jackson St.
Hempstead, N.Y. 11550
Provides information on how to start a mother's center for mutual support.

The Family Resource Coalition
230 North Michigan Avenue, Suite 1625
Chicago, Ill. 60601
Offers a directory of 270 local community resources in 48 states.

The Center for Chinese Medicine
2303 South Garfield Avenue,
Suite 202, Monterey Park, Ca. 91754

The Shiatsu Education Center of America
52 West 55th Street,
New York, N.Y. 10019
Teaches workshops on the Shiatsu (Japanese acupressure) technique for a healthy pregnancy and relief

of pain during childbirth. Book available by mail.

The American Society of Clinical Hypnosis
2250 E. Devon Avenue, Suite 336, Des Plaines
Illinois 60018
A source of information on the use of hypnosis during pregnancy and birth. Send SASE.

IN CASE OF PROBLEMS

The Compassionate Friends
National Headquarters
P.O. Box 1347
Oak Brook, Ill. 60521
A national organization with over 200 chapters devoted to aiding parents in the resolution of grief experienced upon the death of a child.

International Parents' Organization
Alexander Graham Bell Association for the Deaf
3417 Volta Place, N.W.
Washington, D.C. 20007
Offers resources and information for families of hearing-impaired children.

National Sudden Infant Death Syndrome Foundation
Two Metro Plaza (Suite 205)
824- Professional Place
Landover, Md. 20785
Provides information about SIDS and offers support to families who lose young children unexpectedly. Offers referrals to programs at local and state levels.

Further reading

Bernath, Maja. *Parents Book for Your Baby's First Year*, Ballantine Books, 1983.

Bing, Elisabeth. *Six Practical Lessons for an Easier Childbirth*, Bantam Books, 1982.

Bing, Elisabeth and Colman, Libby. *Making Love During Pregnancy*, Bantam Books, 1977.

Bourne, Gordon. *Pregnancy*, Harper & Row, 1974.

Bradley, Robert. *Husband-Coached Childbirth*, third ed., Harper & Row, 1981

Brazelton, T. Berry. *Infants and Mothers: Differences in Development*, rev., Delacorte, 1983.

Brazelton, T. Berry. *On Becoming a Family: The Growth of Attachment*, Delacorte, 1981.

Brewer, Gail, ed. *The Pregnancy after 30 Workbook*, Rodale Press, Inc., 1978.

Caplan, Frank. *The First Twelve Months of Life*, Bantam Books, 1973.

Dale, Barbara and Roeber, Johanna. *The Pregnancy Exercise Book*, Pantheon, 1982.

DeLyser, Femmy. *Jane Fonda's Workout Book for Pregnancy, Birth and Recovery*, Simon & Schuster, 1982.

Henig, Robin Marantz. *Your Premature Baby*, Ballantine Books, 1984.

Keith, Catherine, R.N. and Sperling, Debra, R.N. *The Birthing Book*, Times Books, 1984.

Kitzinger, Sheila. *The Complete Book of Pregnancy and Childbirth*, Knopf, 1980.

LaLeche League. *The Womanly Art of Breastfeeding*, rev., LaLeche League, 1981.

Leach, Penelope. *Your Baby and Child: From Birth to Age Five*, Knopf, 1978.

Lynch-Fraser, Diane. *The Complete Postpartum Guide*, Ballantine Books, 1985.

Nilsson, Linnart. *A Child Is Born*, rev., Delacorte, 1977.

Noble, Elizabeth. *Essential Exercises for the Childbearing Year*, rev., Houghton Mifflin, 1982.

Paulson, Jane Hughes. *Working Pregnant*, Ballantine Books, 1984.

Pryor, Karen. *Nursing Your Baby*, rev., Pocket Books, 1973.

Schrotenboer, Kathryn, OB/GYN and Weiss, Joan Solomon. *The Woman Doctor's Guide to Pregnancy Over 35*, Ballantine Books, 1985.

Spock, Dr. Benjamin. *Baby and Child Care*, rev., Pocket Books, 1976.

Trien, Susan. *Parents Book of Breastfeeding*, Ballantine Books, 1983.

White, Alice. *The Total Nutrition Guide for Mother and Baby: From Pregnancy through the First Three Years*, Ballantine Books, 1983.

Yarrow, Leah. *Parents Book of Pregnancy and Birth*, Ballantine Books, 1984.

Glossary

As far as possible I have made this a non-medical glossary. None of the definitions is full and all of them are biased towards usage in pregnancy.

Abortion The embryo is discarded by the uterus before the 28th week of pregnancy.

Albumin A protein, which if found in the urine of a pregnant woman, can be a sign of pre-eclampsia.

Alpha fetoprotein A substance produced by the fetus. High levels in the mother's blood can indicate neural tube defect or multiple pregnancy.

Alveoli Milk glands in the breast.

Amenorrhoea Temporary or permanent absence of periods.

Amniocentesis A small amount of amniotic fluid is taken from the womb at week 16 to test for fetal defects.

Amniotomy Artificial rupture of the membranes (see p. 188).

Anencephaly A severe congenital abnormality in which the fetus has no brain.

Antibiotics Substances that destroy or reduce the growth of bacteria.

Antibodies Proteins produced by the body to protect it against infection.

Anti-D immunoglobin A special Rhesus antibody injected into a Rhesus negative mother after the birth if any Rhesus positive cells have escaped from her baby into her bloodstream.

Apgar scale or rating Five simple tests to check the baby at birth.

Bag of waters Two thin sheets, the amnion and chorion, line the uterus and form a bag in which the baby develops.

Blastocyst A fertilized egg which is subdivided into groups of cells.

Carpal tunnel syndrome Fluid in the hands during pregnancy. It can cause pressure on the nerves in the wrist, resulting in numbness and tingling in the fingers.

Catheter A tube inserted into the body used to drain the bladder or to introduce fluids.

Cervix The neck of the womb.

Chloasma Discoloration of the skin, often on the face.

Congenital abnormality An abnormality existing at birth which occurred in the womb as a result of drugs, poisons, disease or a damaged gene.

Corpus luteum A glandular mass that forms in the ovary after ovulation and produces progesterone to maintain a pregnancy until week 16 when the placenta takes over.

Crowning When the head can be seen at the vagina.

Diastolic pressure The lower figure in a blood pressure reading.

Doppler A small machine that uses ultrasound to detect the fetal heart *see* **Sonargram**.

Down's syndrome A congenital abnormality caused by a specific gene producing mental handicap.

Eclampsia A rare, more severe form of pre-eclampsia.

Ectopic pregnancy The ovum fails to reach the uterus and grows in the Fallopian tube.

Elective induction Planned induction of labor (see p. 188).

Electronic fetal monitoring Electronic means are used to monitor the fetal heartbeat throughout labor.

Embryo The name given to the fertilized ovum until about week 8.

Enema A fluid introduced into the rectum to empty the bowel.

Engagement The baby's presenting part descends into the pelvic cavity.

Episiotomy Incision made in the perineum to facilitate delivery of the baby.

Estriol Estrogen in the blood or urine, if at low levels in late pregnancy, can indicate that the placenta is not functioning well.

External version (ECV) The attempt to turn the fetus to the cephalic position through abdominal manipulation.

False labor Strong Braxton Hicks contractions near to term that convince the mother she is in labor.

Fetus Name given to the baby in the womb from week 8 until birth.

Fontanelles The soft spots on the baby's skull at birth between unjointed bones.

Fundus The upper part of the uterus.

Hemorrhage Heavy bleeding.

Hormone A substance released by glands which acts as a messenger to stimulate activity in parts of the body.

Human chorionic gonadotrophin (HCG) Causes the ovary to produce more progesterone, thus suppressing menstruation and sustaining the pregnancy. Detection in urine is a reliable pregnancy test.

Hydrocephalus A congenital abnormality of the baby's brain in which the head fills with fluid.

Hypertension High blood pressure.

Hyperventilation Overbreathing or prolonged panting – can cause fainting.

Hypnotic drugs Drugs that induce sleep.

Hypotension Low blood pressure.

Induction Artificial starting of labor by various methods.
Involution of the uterus The process by which the womb returns to normal.
Jaundice Inability of the newborn baby's liver to break down excess red blood cells.
Labia The skin folds at the opening of the vagina.
Lanugo Primitive hair on the body of the fetus in the womb.
Lie The position of the fetus in the womb.
Lightening The time when the baby descends into the pelvic cavity in preparation for birth, also known as engagement.
Linea nigra A darkened line that appears on the abdomen.
Lithotomy position Delivery position in which the woman lies on her back with her feet held in knee braces.
Lochia Discharge from the vagina after delivery.
Meconium The bowel contents of the baby at birth.
Metabolism The process by which the body uses food to grow, keep warm and give energy.
Miscarriage see **Abortion**
Molding The shaping of the presenting part of the baby as it descends the birth canal. Usually the skull, but breech babies have swollen genitals for 24 hours or so.
Monilia Another name for the vaginal infection thrush.
Mucus A sticky substance produced by glands.
Neonatal death When a baby dies within a month of birth.
Neural tube defects (NTD) Abnormalities of the spinal cord, including anencephaly, spina bifida.
Oviduct Another name for the Fallopian tube.
Oxytocin A hormone that causes the uterus to contract and the breasts to make milk.

Pelvic floor The sling of muscles that holds the pelvic organs in place.
Perinatal death Death of the baby within a week of birth.
Perineum The area between the vagina and the rectum.
Pitocin A synthetic form of oxytocin.
Polyhydramnios An excessive amount of amniotic fluid.
Postpartum After the birth.
Pre-eclampsia High blood pressure, retention of fluid and perhaps excess weight can lead to this illness.
Psychoprophylaxis A means of preparation for childbirth by preparing your mind.
Puerperium The period of 4–6 weeks after delivery.
Pyelonephritis Infection of the kidneys.
Pyridoxine Vitamin B6.
Sedative A drug that calms and induces sleepiness.
Shirodkar The purse-string suture inserted into an incompetent cervix.
Show Blood-stained mucus from the vagina indicating that the cervix is dilating and labor is about to begin.
Sonargram The use of ultrasound to listen to the fetal heartbeat.
Speculum A duck-billed metal instrument inserted into the vagina so that the doctor can see the cervix.
Sphincter A muscle controlling an opening.
Stethoscope, fetal A trumpet-shaped hearing device to detect the fetal heart. It is placed against the mother's abdomen.
Stillbirth The fetus is discarded from the womb after the 28th week.
Stress incontinence Involuntary leakage of urine resulting from weakness in the pelvic floor muscles when abdominal pressure increases.

Stress tests Inducing contractions during late pregnancy to evaluate the fetus' ability to tolerate labor itself.
Suture Surgical stitch.
Symphysis pubis The point at which the two pubic bones are joined.
Systolic pressure The top figure in a blood pressure reading; taken when the heart contracts and pumps blood.
Test weighing Weighing the baby before and after a breastfeeding to check on the amount of breast milk taken.
Tochodynamometer A monitor on a belt attached to the mother's abdomen during labor to record contractions.
Toxemia Another term for pre-eclampsia (see p. 150).
Toxoplasmosis, congenital This is a rare, parasitic disease that can cause blindness in the fetus. It is carried by cat faeces.
Transducer The instrument that tracks across the abdomen during a scan.
Trial of labor The early part of a labor which is planned to go to Cesarean section; used to test whether a vaginal delivery may prove possible.
Trimester One third of a pregnancy.
Urethra The canal that carries urine from the bladder.
Uterine inertia The failure of the uterus to contract strongly enough for labor to proceed.
Vernix A white substance that covers the fetus in the uterus to protect it from becoming soggy in the amniotic fluid.
Viability The baby's ability to survive after birth. A fetus is viable in law at week 28 of pregnancy.
Wharton's jelly The substance that surrounds the blood vessels making up the umbilical cord.

Index

A

Abdominal exercise 116
  postnatal 216–17
Abdominal pain 136–7
Abdominal palpation 61
Abnormal babies
  alcohol and 24
  diet of mother and 22, 96
  Down's syndrome 24, 29, 68
  genetic counselling and 29
  hazards at work and 33
  marijuana and 23
  miscarriage of 149
  prenatal screening 67–9
  rubella effects in 24
  smoking and 105
  socio-economic state and 22, 24
ABO blood group 61
Abortion
  induced 148
  spontaneous (miscarriage) 33, 81, 95, 146, 148–9
Aches 87, 108
Acne 126, 127
Acupuncture 185
Afterpains of uterus 207
Age of parents 24, 32
Alcohol and abnormality 24, 106–7
Alpha fetoprotein (AFP) screening 61, 64, 69
Alternative birthing room 54
Amenorrhoea (missed period) 35
Amniocentesis 68–9
Amniotic fluid 68, 70–1
  meconium in 197
Amniotomy 188
Analgesics in labor 50, 183–6
Anemia 61, 86
  iron-deficiency 86, 144
Ankle exercises 117, 216
Anus, anal sphincter 112
Anxiety see **Fears**
Apgar scale in newborn 206
Appearance 122–7
Arm exercises 114, 115
Areola 82–3, 88
Artificial insemination (AID, AIH) 33

B

Baby, newborn
  Apgar scale of 206
  bathing 212
  birth 174–6
  birthweight 199
  blood transfusion 151
  bonding with mother 56, 202–4, 215
  breathing at birth 50, 206
  burping 210
  changing 212–13
  check-up 224
  childcarers for 40–1, 224–5
  children (siblings) and 205, 219–20, 221
  clothes 155, 157
  crying 226
  diapers 154, 212–13
  drugs at birth and 182, 186
  equipment 152–5
  father and 220–1
  feeding times 218–19
  feeding 208–11
  first days 202–15
  hearing acuteness 50
  heat loss at birth 50
  jaundice in 198
  Leboyer birth ideas 49–50
  newborn reflexes 206
  nursery for 152
  postmature 189
  postnatal checks 206, 215
  premature 199–200
  preparing home for 152–3
  routine for 204–5, 218–19
  spitting up 210
  stillborn 200–1
  topping and tailing 212–13
  see also **Abnormal babies, Fetus**
Back
  exercises 117
  movements in pregnancy 109
Back labor 160, 161
Backache 87, 136–7
Bassinets 153
Bed
  in childbirth 52
  in home birth 156
Bending 109
Birth see **Childbirth**
Birth assistant 10, 47–8
  aids for 157
  countdown for labor and 159
  in first stage 166
  in second stage 172
  in transition 169
Birth defects see **Abnormal babies**
Birthing centers 43
Birthing stools 52
Bladder
  infection 142–3
  pain after birth 224
  in pregnancy 87
Blastocyst formation 13, 30
Bleeding
  breakthrough, in early pregnancy 81
  gums 136–7
  in miscarriage 148–9
  postnatal 107, 198–9
  sex and 95

  third trimester 144–5
Blood
  alpha fetoprotein (AFP) 61, 67, 69
  groups 61, 150–1
  prenatal tests 61, 62, 63
  RH groups 150–1
  types and miscarriage 148
  volume in pregnancy 86
Blood pressure
  high (hypertension) 61, 146, 150
  postnatal check 224
  prenatal checks 61, 63
Body
  care of 122, 126–7
  changes to 80–9, 108
  see also **Exercises, Health**
Bonding 202–4, 215
  breastfeeding and 56
Bottle feeding 57, 210–11
Bottom exercise 117
Bowels after birth 207, 224
Boy, to conceive 29
Brain abnormality,
  screening of fetus 67
Braces, knee 53–4
Bras
  nursing (maternity) 83, 127, 210
  pregnancy 83, 127
Braxton Hicks contractions 85, 159, 161
Breasts
  breastfeeding and 56, 83, 210
  change in pregnancy 35, 82–3
  engorgement 210
  exercise for 116
  hormone effects on 82
  lactating 83
  in menstrual cycle 81
  nipples 35, 60, 82, 83, 88
  prenatal check 60
Breastfeeding 55–7, 208–10
  advantages and
    disadvantages 55–7
  bras for 83, 127, 210
  contraception and 223
  diet and 221
  getting going 209, 210
  let-down reflex 203, 209
  nipples and 60, 83, 209, 210
  outside work and 224–5
Breast milk
  analysis of 56
  disease protection 55
  expression and storage 56–7, 200, 210, 224–5
  in pregnancy 104
  see also **Colostrum**
Breast pads 127, 210
Breast reliever 224
Breast shield 60, 83
Breathing techniques 132, 163
Breathlessness 140–1
Breech birth 192
Breech presentation, twins 147
Brown pigment 82, 83, 88

C

Calcium 101, 103
Carriages 154
Cephalic presentation,
  twins 147
Cervical cap, contraceptive 223,
  224
Cervix 86
  cervical smears 60, 224
  erosion 136–7
  in labor 86, 164
  incompetent 146
Cesarean section 193–7
  breech birth and 192
  elective 193
  epidural in 194, 195
  reasons for 197
Chest exercise 115
Childbirth and labor
  aids for 157
  baby's head in 112, 113
  birth assistant and 10, 47, 157,
    159, 160–91
  birth of baby 174–6
  breech birth 148
  choices in 42–57
  complications in 192–201
  countdown for 159
  early signs 159
  false labor 85
  first stage 164–8
  food and drink in 54
  at home 44–5, 159
  in the hospital 46–8, 51–4, 159
  intercourse and 95
  internal examination in 165
  induction of 188–9
  length of 161
  medical intervention in 186–91
  natural 49–51
  onset of 161
  pain and pain relief in 160–1,
    182–6
  positions for 44, 50–4, 119,
    168–71
  pre-labor 160, 161
  preparation 156–9
  procedures in 51–4
  second stage 171, 172–81
  sudden delivery 181
  transitional stage 169–71
  twins 181
Childcarers for baby 40–1,
  224–5
Children (siblings)
  baby and 205, 219–20, 221
  during the hospital stay 158–9
Chloasma 126
Chorionic villi 81, 82
Chromosomes 28
  counts and abnormality 29,
    68–9
  damage and smoking 23
  sex 28, 29
Cigarettes see Smoking

Classes, prenatal 62, 64
  exercises 110, 111
  infantcare 64
Clinics, prenatal 58, 59, 62
Clothes
  for baby 155, 157
  for birth 157
  in pregnancy 122–5
Colostrum 202, 208, 209
  importance for baby 55, 208,
    209
  in pregnancy 82, 83
Complete abortion 149
Conception 22–33
Condom 223
Congenital malformations
  see Abnormal babies
Constipation 82, 136–7
Contraception, postnatal 215,
  223, 224
Contractions 94, 207
  Braxton-Hicks 85, 159, 161
  breathing during 132
  false labor 85
  at labor onset 160–1
  in labor 161, 190–1
  postnatal 202
  pushing out baby 172–4
  in transition 169
Corpus luteum 80–1
Costal margin pain 140–1
Cows' milk allergy 57
Cramps 136–7
Cravings 35, 136–7
Cribs 153
Crying baby 226
Cystitis 142–3

D

Delivery see Childbirth and
  labor
Delivery room 54, 64
Demerol 183, 186
Depression
  miscarriage and 149
  postpartum blues 214–15
  in pregnancy 90
Diabetes 60, 145
Diapers 154
  changing 212–13
Dick-Read, Grantley, and
  natural childbirth 49
Diet see Nutrition
Dilation of cervix 86, 164
Dilation and curettage 149
Discomfort in bed 136–7
Doctor 43
  home birth and 43, 44, 62
  obstetrician 43, 48, 62
  prenatal care by 58, 62
Dominant characteristics
  inheritance of 28
Douche, vaginal, and sex of
  baby 29

Down's syndrome
  amniocentesis check 68–9
  genetic counselling 29
  mother's age and 24
Dreams 93–4
Drugs
  conception and 23–4, 25
  in labor 50, 182–6
  in pregnancy 106–7

E

Ectopic pregnancy 145
Edema 60, 138
Effacement of cervix 164
Egg see Ovum
Ejaculation and sperm 30, 31
Elderly primipara 10, 64; see also
  Amniocentesis, Older mother
Electronic fetal monitoring
  (EFM) 162, 190–1
Embryo 13–14, 30, 31, 81
  development 72
Emotional changes 90–5
Emotions and hormones 90
Endometrium (uterus lining) 80,
  81
Enemas before birth 51
Engagement of head in
  pelvis 65, 159
Epidural anesthetic 187
Episiotomy 186–7
  hair shaving and 52
Estimated date of confinement
  (EDC) 12, 66–7, 189
  calculation of 37
  fundus height and 61, 65, 85
Estrogen 80, 81
  breast effects 82, 83
  in early pregnancy 35
  placental production 82
Exercise 108–21
  before conception 23
  sports 120–1
Exercises
  Kegel 112–13
  pelvic floor 112–13
  pelvis 118–19
  postnatal 216–17
  prenatal classes 110, 111
  routines 110
  warm-up 114–15
  water 121
External cephalic
  version (ECV) 61, 192
Eye color genes 28
Eyes 142–3

F

Fainting 138–9

Fallopian tubes
blockages 32
ectopic pregnancy in 145
egg movement down 80
fertilization in 30–1
False labor 85
Family
home birth and 44, 45
routine after birth 218–19
see also **Children, Father**
Father/Partner 10, 25
baby and 220–1
as birth assistant 47–8
blood group incompatibility 61, 68, 148, 150
bonding with baby 202, 204
bottle feeding by 57, 210–11
Cesarean section and 194
children and 159
feelings in pregnancy 92
health, pre-conception 29
labor aids for 157
labor countdown and 159
labor help 166, 169, 172
postnatal role 220–1
in pregnancy 92, 93
relaxation help 131, 133
sex after birth 222–3
stillbirth and 200, 201
working mother and 40
see also **Birth Assistant**
Fears and anxieties
after miscarriage 149
in pregnancy 25, 90, 93–4
Feeding 55–7, 208–11
bottle feeding 57, 210–11
breastfeeding 55–7, 208–10
routines 204, 218–19
Female, to conceive 29
Fertility and infertility
age and 24, 32
low 32–3
smoking and 23
work hazards and 33
Fertilization 30–3, 80
Fetoscopy 67, 162
Fetus 31
age determination 66–7
birth preparation for 112, 113
"dips" of heartbeat 190–1
distress in labor 197
electronic fetal monitoring (EFM) 162, 190–1
growth 14–21, 60, 67, 70–9
head engagement 159
heartbeat 61, 162, 190–1
lack of movement of 145
lie in uterus 61, 65, 161
miscarriage 148, 149
RH blood group 150–1
smoking and 105
ultrasound scan 66–7
see also **Abnormal babies**
Fever in late pregnancy 145
Fiber 100
Fitness *see* **Health and Fitness**
Flatulence 138–9
Fluid intake 100

Fluid retention 60, 63, 88
pre-eclampsia and 150
Folic acid 61, 87, 102, 103
Follicle, ovarian 80
Follicle-stimulating hormone (FSH) 30, 80
Food *see* **Nutrition**
Food cravings 35
Foot exercises 115, 117, 216
Footwear 124
Forceps delivery 197–8
Fundus height 61, 65, 85

G

Genes, influence of 28
Genetic counselling 29
Genetic diseases, amniocentesis check 68. 69
Genital herpes 60
German measles (rubella) infection 24, 61, 215
Gingivitis 136–7
Girl, to conceive 29
Gums 89, 136–7

H

Habitual abortion 149
Hair color genes 28
Hair 89, 126
Hand exercises 114
Hemoglobin 61, 86
Hemophilia and genetic counselling 29
Hemorrhage
postpartum 198–9
third trimester 144–5
Head exercise 117
Headache in late pregnancy 145
Health and fitness
after childbirth 40
exercises for 108–21
postnatal 216–17
pre-conception 22–3, 108
in pregnancy 60–1, 96–105, 108, 110
Heart
fetal and newborn 61, 206
maternal 86, 146
Heartburn 138–9
Height of mother 60
High blood pressure (hypertension) in pregnancy 61, 146
pre-eclampsia and 150
Hip exercise 116
Home
delivery 43, 44–5, 62, 156–7, 159
preparing for baby 152–3
routine after birth 218–19

Hormones
estrogen 35, 80–3
follicle-stimulating hormone (FSH) 30, 80
human chorionic gonadotrophin (HCG) 34, 35, 80–1, 82
human placental lactogen (HPL) 82
melanocyte stimulating hormone (MSH) 82
miscarriage and 148
mood changes and 90
ovarian 80, 82
oxytocin 209
pituitary 80
placental 80–2
in pregnancy 34–5, 80–3
progesterone 34–5, 80–3, 112
relaxin 82
therapy for infertility 32–3
Hospital
admission procedure 162
alternative birthing room 54
birth 43, 46–8, 51–4, 156–9
delivery room 54
discharge 215
maternity units 43, 215
what to take 157
Human chorionic gonadotrophin (HCG) 34, 35, 80–1, 82
Human placental lactogen (HPL) 82
Hypertension *see* **High blood pressure**
Hypnosis 185

I

Immunization
for baby 224
rubella 24, 61, 215
Implantation of embryo 30–1, 80
Incompetent cervix 146
Incomplete abortion 149
Incontinence, urinary 112, 138–9
Incubators 200
Induction of labor 188–9
Inevitable abortion 149
Infections, sex and 94, 95
Infertility *see* **Fertility and infertility**
Injections, contraceptive 223
Insomnia 128, 138–9
Intelligence and parental bonding 204
Internal examination
in labor 165
in pregnancy 36, 60
Intra-uterine device (IUD) 223, 224
ectopic pregnancy and 145
Intrauterine transfusion 151
Iron 86, 101–2, 103
supplements 61, 62, 102, 144

J

Jaundice of newborn 151, 198
Joints 87, 108

K

Kegel exercises 112–13
Kidneys 87
  damage 150
  infection 60
Kitzinger, Sheila,
  episiotomy survey 187

L

Labor see Childbirth and
  Labor
Lactation see Breasts,
  Breastfeeding
Lamaze, Fernand, natural
  childbirth method 49
Lanugo 74
Laproscopy and infertility 32
Leboyer, Frederick, philosophy
  of 49–50
Leg exercises 115
Let-down reflex 209
Lifting 109
Ligaments 87, 108
Linea nigra 88
Lithotomy position 54
Lochia, postnatal 198–9, 207
Looks 122–7
Lungs 87

M

Make up 126, 127
Male, to conceive 29
Malformations see Abnormal
  babies
Marijuana and abnormality 23
Massage 133
Maternal bonding 202–4, 215
Maternity centers 43
McDonald suture 146
Meconium in amniotic fluid 197
Melanocyte stimulating
  hormone (MSH) 82
Membrane rupture 145, 161
  artificial (amniotomy,
    ARM) 188
Membranes 70–1
Meningitis in baby and herpes
  infection 60
Menstrual cycle 30, 80, 81, 82

Menstruation
  after childbirth 40
  confinement date (EDC) and 57
  missed period
    (amenorrhoea) 35
  suppression in pregnancy 80–2
Metabolic disease, amniocentesis
  and 69
Metabolism 128
Micturition see Urination
Milk see Breast milk, Colostrum,
  Cow's milk
Minerals 87, 101–3; see also Iron
Miscarriage 33, 81, 148–9
  incompetent cervix and 146
  intercourse and 95
  threatened 148, 149
  types 149
  what to do 148
Missed abortion 149
Mongol babies see Down's
  syndrome
Monthly cycle 30, 80, 81, 82
Monitoring
  electronic fetal monitoring
    (EFM) 162, 190–1
  telemetry 191
Morning sickness 35, 82, 104,
  138–9
  and diet 104
Moro reflex 206
Movements
  baby's 74, 145
  mother's 108–9
Multiple pregnancy 147
  hormone therapy and 33
  ultrasound detection 67
  see also Twins
Muscles 108

N

Nails 89
Nasal discomfort 138–9
Nausea 35, 82, 104, 145
  diet and 104
Neck exercise 117
Neural tube defects, screening
  for 67
Nipples
  colour 82, 88
  feeding and 209, 210
  inverted or flat 60, 83
  in pregnancy 35, 82, 83, 88
Nurse Midwife 43, 48, 62
Nursery and equipment 152–5
Nutrition of mother
  foods to avoid 98, 99
  miscarriage and 148
  morning sickness and 104
  postnatal 221
  pre-conception 22
  in pregnancy 60, 87, 89, 96–105
  vital nutrients 100–3
  vulnerable women and 101

O

Obesity 98
Obstetricians 43, 48, 62
Odent, Michel, ideas of 50–1,
  111
Older mothers 10, 24
  amniocentesis for 68, 69
  prenatal care 64
Ovaries
  hormones from 80, 82
  ovarian cycle 30
Ovulation 30, 80
  hormone therapy for 32–3
  infertility and 32
Ovum (egg)
  chromosomes and genes 28, 29
  ectopic pregnancy of 145
  fertilization 30–3, 80–1
  healthy or defective 29
Oxytocin 209
  -induced labor 188–9

P

Pain
  in pregnancy 87, 108
  and relief in labor 50, 182–6
Palpation, abdominal 61
Parents
  bonding with baby 204, 215
  parentcraft classes 62, 64
  parenthood and lifestyle 25
  recognition by baby 40–1
Partner see Father/Partner
Pectoral exercises 116
Pelvic floor exercises 112–13,
  118–19, 216
Pelvic floor muscles 112–13
Pelvis
  brim 65
  discomfort 140–1
  engagement of head in 65, 159
  internal examination 60
  ligament elasticity 87
  pelvic outlet 60
  pelvic tilt 87, 118
  presentation of baby and 65
  size 60
Perineum, episiotomy and 186–7
Periods see Menstruation
Phototherapy for jaundice 198
Pigmentation 82, 83, 88, 140–1
  skin care and 126
Piles 140–1
Pill, contraceptive 223
Pituitary gland 80
Placenta 30, 31, 70–1, 81, 82
  hormones from 80–2
  miscarriage and 148, 149
  postnatal retention 198–9
  ultrasound scan 66–7, 144
Placenta abruptio 144

Placenta previa 95, 144–5
Placental insufficiency 148, 150, 189, 200
Planning a baby 22–33
Positions in labor 44, 52
  on back 52, 53–4
  in back labor 169
  for delivery 52–3, 171
  first stage 168
  at Odent clinic 50–1
  squatting 50–1, 171
  transition 170
  upright 52, 53
Postmaturity, signs of 189
Postnatal period 202–17
  check-up 215, 224
  exercises 216–17
  first days 202–17
  normal routine 218–27
  postpartum blues 214–15
  see also **Baby**
Postpartum blues 214–15
Postpartum hemorrhage 198–9
Posture in pregnancy 108, 109
Potatoes as food source 104
Pre-eclamptic toxemia (PET)
  prenatal tests 60, 61
  signs of 146, 150
Pregnancy
  confirmation 34–41, 58, 60
  duration 12
  early symptoms 12, 34–5
  feelings about 34, 36–7
  physical changes 12–21, 80–9
  tests 12, 36, 82
  working woman and 38–41
  see also **Conception, Estimated date of confinement (EDC), Prenatal care**
Premature baby 199–200
  forceps delivery 197–8
Prenatal care 58–69
  abbreviations used in 65
  classes 62, 64, 110, 111
  clinics 36, 58, 59, 62
  doctor and 58, 59
  exercise class 110, 111
  routine tests 60–1
  special tests 66–9
  see also **Pregnancy**
Presentation of baby 65, 161
  breech 147–8, 192
  cephalic 65
  external cephalic version (ECV) 61, 192
  twins 147
Progesterone 80, 81, 82
  breast effects 82, 83
  in early pregnancy 34–5
  placental production 82
  softening effect 112
Prolapse of uterus 112
Prostaglandin suppositories 188
Protein–rich foods 100
Protein in urine 60
Psychoprophylaxis, natural childbirth method 49
Pubic hair shaving 51–2

R

Rashes 140–1
Recessive characteristics 28
Recurrent abortion 149
Reflexes of newborn 206
Relaxation and rest
  partner's help 131, 133
  postnatal 214, 221
  in pregnancy 34–5, 128–35
  techniques 17, 130–1
  tiredness 142–3
Relaxin, effects 82
RH blood groups 61, 150–1
  incompatibility 61, 68, 150
  RH negative mothers 150–1
Rib pain 140–1
Rooting reflex 209, 211
Round ligament pain 136–7
Rubella (German measles) infection 24, 61, 215
Rupture of membranes 145, 161

S

Sacroiliac joint 87
  pain 136–7
Salpingitis, coil-induced 145
Salt and sodium 81, 86, 99, 103
Self-image 90–1, 122
Sex determination of baby 28–9
Sex-linked disorders
  amniocentesis checks 68, 69
Sex
  after birth 222–3
  in pregnancy 94–5
  sperm and 29, 30, 31
Shaving of pubic hair 51–2
Shirodkar suture 146
Shoes 125
Shoulder exercises 115, 117
Show, at labor onset 161
Siblings see **Children**
Sitting exercises 109, 117
Sickle cell disease 61
Single parenthood by choice 25
Skin 87, 88, 122, 126
  care and make-up 126, 127
  pigmentation 82, 83, 88, 126, 140–1
  stretch marks 88, 140–1
Sleep
  postnatal period 214
  in pregnancy 128–9
Smoking 23
  effects 23, 148
  pre-conception 23
  in pregnancy 105
  to cut down 105
Social factors 22, 24, 148
Sodium see **Salt**
Sperm
  fertilization 30–1

  genetics 28, 29
  healthy or defective 23, 29
  infertility and 32, 33
  sex and 28, 29
Sphincter muscles 112
Spider veins 126
Spina bifida screening 67, 68, 69
Spine movements 109
  exercises 117
Spontaneous abortion see **Miscarriage**
Sports 120–1
Squatting
  birth position 50–1, 171
  exercises 119
Stillbirth 200–1
Stitches
  coping with 207
  episiotomy and 186–7
Stretchmarks 88, 140–1
Strollers 154
Sweating 140–1
Swelling 145, 150
Swimming 120, 121
Syphilis, prenatal tests 61

T

Taste changes 142–3
Tearing, avoidance in labor 112, 113
Teeth 89
Telemetry 191
Tension relaxation techniques 117, 130–1
Thalassemia 61
Thigh exercises 116, 117
Third trimester bleeding 144–5
Threatened abortion 148, 149
Thrush 142–3
Tiredness see **Relaxation**
Toxemia see **Pre-eclamptic toxemia**
Transitional stage of labor 169–71
  breathing during 132
  positions in 170
Trial of labor 193
Trimester growth of fetus 72–9
Twins 147
  birth 181
  conception 31
  detection 67, 147
  presentation 147
  types 31, 147

U

Ultrasound scans 66–7, 144
Umbilical cord 215
Urethra 112
Urinary incontinence 112

Urinary tract infection 142–3
Urination (micturition)
  after delivery 207
  in pregnancy 35, 138–9, 145,
  159
Urine
  pregnancy tests 36, 82
  prenatal tests 60, 62, 63
  protein in 150
  sugar in 145
Uterus (womb)
  after birth 224
  afterpains 207
  birth position and 52–3
  endometrium (lining) 80, 81
  expansion 84
  fibroid tumours in 148
  fundus height 61, 65, 85
  implantation in 30–1, 80
  internal examination of 36, 60
  lie of the fetus in 61, 65
  lochia, postnatal 198–9, 207
  miscarriage and 148, 149
  muscles 84, 94
  postpartum hemorrhage 198–9
  in pregnancy 84–6
  prolapse 112
  see also **Contractions, Fetus,**
    Placenta

Working women
  childcarers and 40–1, 225
  hazards and 33, 148
  mothers 10, 25, 40–1, 224–5
  in pregnancy 38–9
  rights and benefits 232–3
Wrist exercises 114

X

X chromosome 28, 29

Y

Y chromosome 28, 29
Yoga 111
  yogic childbirth method 51

Z

Zinc 103

V

Vaccination see **Immunization**
Vacuum extraction
  (ventouse) 201
Vagina 30, 86, 112
  bleeding from 144–5, 148, 149
  douching and sex of baby 29
  infection 142–3
  internal examination and 36
  secretions 32, 86, 142–3, 159
  sex after birth and 222, 223
  sphincter muscles 112
Varicose veins 60, 142–3
Vegetarian diet 100
Vein problems 60, 126
Ventouse (vacuum
  extraction) 201
Vernix 75, 79
Visual disturbances 142–3
Vitamins 87, 101, 102
Vomiting 35, 145

W

Waist exercise 114
Water exercises 120, 121
Weight
  excess 98, 150
  postnatal 55–6
  in pregnancy 60, 63, 96–9
Womb see **Uterus**

Acknowledgments

Dorling Kindersley would like to thank the following for their help in the presentation of this book: Ann Burnham, Polly Dawes, Anne Fisher and Jane Tetzlaff for design help; Ken Hone and Gene Nocon for their photographic services; Sue Brinkhurst, Jean Coombes, Bill and Lizzie Frizzell, Sally Godfrey, Margaret Gold, Sarah Judah, Katie Reed and Monica Reed for being models for the reference shots; The Dance Centre and Pineapple Studios, Covent Garden, and Mothercare for lending clothes; and Paul Stannard from the Charing Cross Hospital for checking the artwork. The photographer and the publishers would also like to thank those parents who allowed us to photograph their pregnancies and labors for this book, and the staff at the Royal Free Hospital, Hampstead, and St. Thomas' Hospital, Lambeth, London.

Additional photography
Jan Baldwin (pp. 114–115; 116–117; 118; 216–217)

Illustration
Edwina Keene
Jenny Powell
David Lawrence
Kuo Kang Chen
Coral Mula

Index
Anne Hardy

Typesetting
Tradespools Limited,
Frome, Somerset.

Reproduction
Repro Llovet, Barcelona

Author's acknowledgments
I am indebted to my editor Charyn Jones whose thoroughness and intelligence, coupled with sheer good humor, is unique in my experience. Gillian Della Casa has designed the book with great flair and creativeness and equally I owe her my gratitude.

Editor Charyn Jones
Art Editor Gillian Della Casa
Senior Art Editor Anne-Marie Bulat
Managing Editor Daphne Razazan

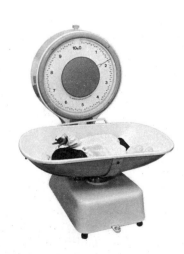